massage for
health

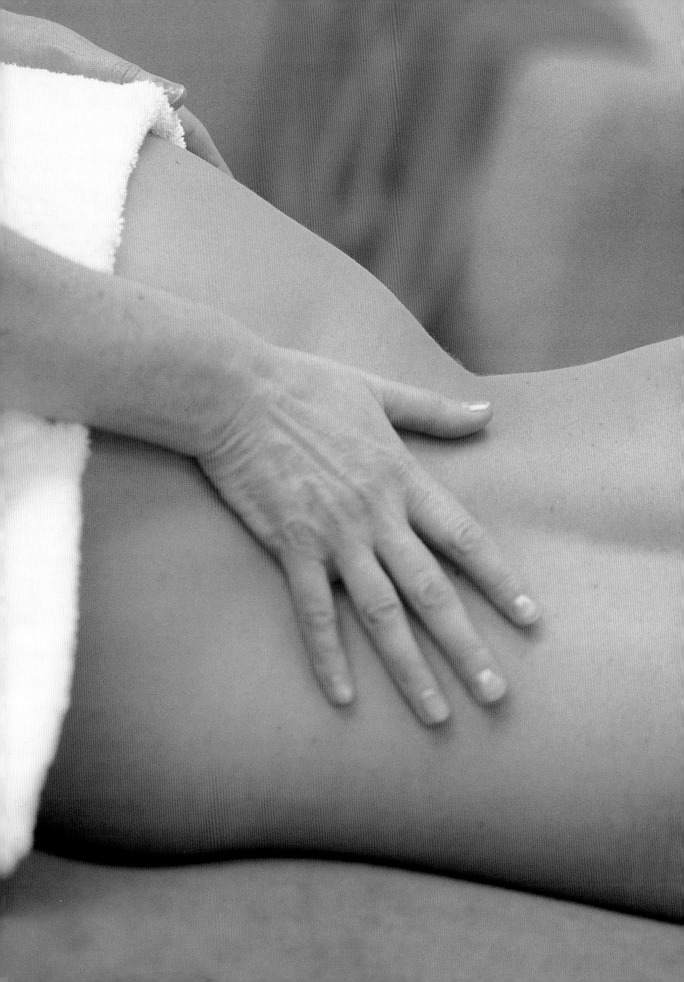

Susan Mumford

hamlyn

Warning: Massage should not be considered as a replacement for professional medical treatment; a physician should be consulted in all matters relating to health and especially in relation to any symptoms which may require diagnosis or medical attention. Care should be taken during pregnancy, particularly in the use of essential oils and pressure points. For babies and children, only use gentle effleurage strokes for a few minutes at a time. For further advice see Contraindications in How To Use This Book.

how to use this book

I have divided this book into six main sections. The Introduction provides an explanation to the concept of energy as a healing force and shows how it has been used throughout the ages and by many different cultures to promote harmony of mind and body. I have also included my thoughts on what it takes to be healer, an ability we all have within us.

In the second section, Healing Techniques, I have explained the various healing techniques we can use, both on and off the body. This predominantly involves sensing but I have also included the important aspects of giving, connecting, balancing and releasing.

My third section, Massage Techniques, provides a step-by-step guide to the various massage strokes and pressures you will need for a healing massage. This section opens with the techniques most commonly used. The strokes featured in both the second and third sections should be used in conjunction with the fourth section, Healing Massage, which shows how to do round-the-body massage and includes an explanation of how to apply the relevant strokes. This massage will release, relax and restore balance within the body. It is within this fourth section that directional guidelines first appear. The dotted line represents a broad guideline for healing techniques, indicating the way in which the giver should direct his attention. The solid line represents the direction that the massage strokes should take.

The fifth section, Common Ailments, shows you how to treat various common ailments such as headaches, menstrual problems, joint and muscle conditions and circulatory, respiratory and digestive complaints. This section includes step-by-step sequences for massaging the affected parts of the body. I have also included some personal anecdotes of my healing experiences with various clients.

The last section, Self Healing, is concerned with how you can take care of yourself. All too often we are so busy concentrating on other people that we forget about our own needs. Relaxing and balancing the mind and body, as well as generally caring for yourself and your spiritual needs, are important aspects of healing.

While you do not need medical qualifications to massage, and while the sensitivity of your hands guides your strokes, it is useful to have as a reference point a basic knowledge of the musculo-skeletal structure beneath your hands. These pages show diagrams of the skeleton and superficial muscles. In this massage, the muscles of the back are particularly important. The trapezius in the upper back, which stretches across the shoulders, nearly always needs attention. In addition, latissimus dorsi and the gluteal muscles usually need to be relaxed. The spine is of great importance to the massage, in particular, the vertebrae of the neck, upper back and sacrum. It is also helpful to be aware of the range of movement of the joints.

the skeleton

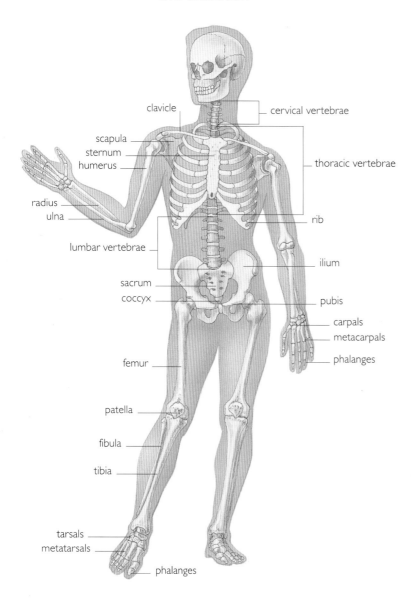

- clavicle
- cervical vertebrae
- scapula
- sternum
- humerus
- thoracic vertebrae
- radius
- ulna
- lumbar vertebrae
- rib
- ilium
- sacrum
- coccyx
- pubis
- carpals
- metacarpals
- phalanges
- femur
- patella
- fibula
- tibia
- tarsals
- metatarsals
- phalanges

Contraindications

If you give massage:

o Make sure that you use light pressure only during pregnancy. Do not massage over the abdomen during the first four months of pregnancy.

o Only use gentle effleurage strokes on babies and children.

o Do not massage over varicose veins, cuts, recent injuries or scar tissue, swelling, tumours, rashes or infected areas.

o Always seek medical approval in cases of heart condition.

o Medical advice to be sought if acute pain is experienced during massage.

If you receive massage:

o Advise if you are pregnant.

o Avoid a heavy meal two hours beforehand.

o Avoid alcohol six hours before and after the massage.

These techniques are intended as a guide and are not a substitute for professional training or medical help.

Massage tips

Preparing for massage:

o The massage environment should be warm and relaxing.

o Carry out the massage on a firm and comfortable surface.

o Remove any jewellery and ensure your nails are short.

o Refer back to the techniques section throughout the round-the-body massage.

o Wash your hands before and after each massage.

o Try both the healing and the massage techniques on yourself before using them on a partner.

The massage:

o Set aside approximately 45–60 minutes for a session.

o Use a few drops of grapeseed or sweet almond oil.

o Repeat each stroke several times, unless told otherwise.

After the massage:

o Carry out the cleansing techniques on yourself.

o Treat any confidences with the greatest respect.

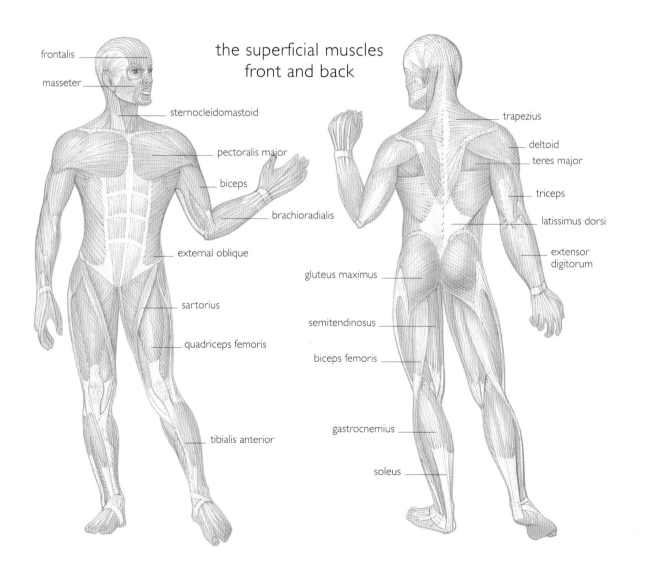

the superficial muscles front and back

frontalis
masseter
sternocleidomastoid
pectoralis major
biceps
brachioradialis
external oblique
sartorius
quadriceps femoris
tibialis anterior

trapezius
deltoid
teres major
triceps
latissimus dorsi
extensor digitorum
gluteus maximus
semitendinosus
biceps femoris
gastrocnemius
soleus

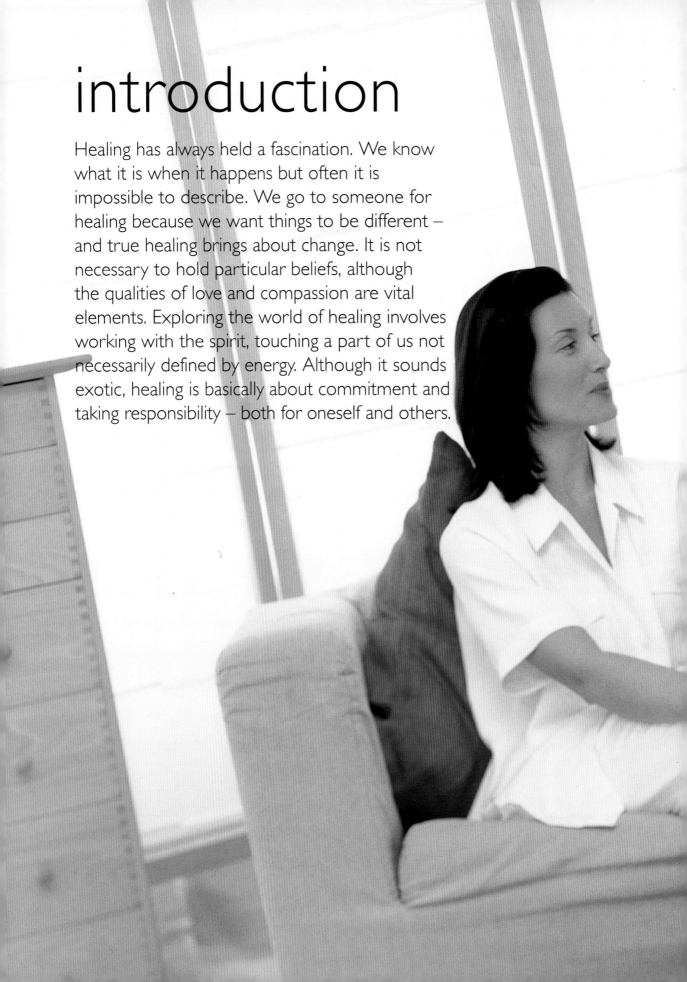

introduction

Healing has always held a fascination. We know what it is when it happens but often it is impossible to describe. We go to someone for healing because we want things to be different – and true healing brings about change. It is not necessary to hold particular beliefs, although the qualities of love and compassion are vital elements. Exploring the world of healing involves working with the spirit, touching a part of us not necessarily defined by energy. Although it sounds exotic, healing is basically about commitment and taking responsibility – both for oneself and others.

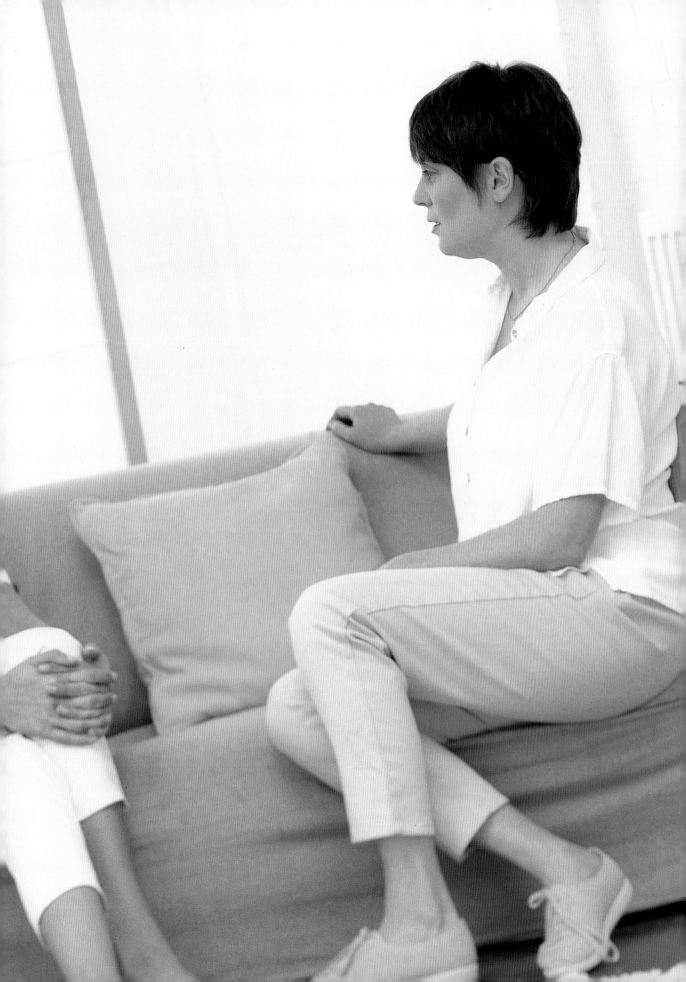

what is healing?

The dictionary gives a good definition of healing: to restore to health or to cure. The healing process can be prompted by many things: orthodox medicines, herbal remedies, physical and mental therapies, rest, nutrition, new interests, relationships and love. Any of these methods can tip the balance and restore us to health.

Illness occurs when all the varying aspects of ourselves are not in harmony and energy is not nourishing our body. We need to be in balance. Neglecting our emotional or spiritual sides may result in disease in the same way as neglecting our bodies results in physical deterioration.

However, illness, disease and death are part of life. Some see illness as positive, providing an opportunity to resolve some past conflict so that they can move on. Oddly enough, illness may be just what one needs to bring about change. It can be a time of transition and a time to reflect. Illness focuses the attention, precipitating crisis and initiating a re-evaluation of ourselves. Some people say illness is the best thing that has ever happened to them, so it is not the healer's role to take away the positive aspects of this experience.

The form of healing we are looking at in this book is perhaps the most traditional image – working to restore health in a non-invasive way. Usually, healing is given through the hands, which are placed gently on the body or held slightly away. The receiver may feel a range of sensations, from slight tingling, currents or waves, to a pleasant feeling of relaxation and well-being. The intention of healing is to bring about change. The body and physical illness are linked to the mind, emotions, energy and spirit. It is a dynamic relationship involving an exchange. It is a sending of energies from healer to receiver – like recharging a battery. The healer will use his or her sensitivity to gain an impression of the receiver's condition. What appears to take place is a replenishment of the receiver's energies, enabling the receiver to heal him- or herself, so while the healer is the initiator of the healing process, self-healing is what eventually occurs.

Healing is not an intellectual process and is therefore difficult to describe. The dynamic relationship between the healer and receiver is of paramount importance. For healing to take place there needs to be willingness on both sides. There are many discussions about the different methods used and it would be wrong to say that one is better than another.

Many think healing is synonymous with religion, while others are put off by the word 'spiritual'. However, the best form of healing comes not from the healer's own energy but from some source outside.

what is energy?

Energy makes up our universe and is a term used to describe activity. Energy is all around us. It comes from the ground, is in the atmosphere, circulates in our bodies and loops round our bones. In short, everything is made up of energy, and has its own distinct patterns.

We are exchanging energy all the time. As we now know from scientific discovery, the universe is not made up of solid objects existing independently in empty space. It is composed of complex, ever-changing patterns of interactions. Each thing that exists does not exist in isolation but forms part of a pattern of relationships that make up the whole. Indeed, its very nature is defined by the way it interacts with its environment. Each thing can only be understood in terms of its relationships.

As we now also know, mass is not solid but is a form of energy – and that energy is dynamic. It is constantly interacting to form new patterns and relationships which last for varying lengths of time. Nothing is static, all is constantly changing. So how does this help us to understand ourselves and the interaction which forms a vital part of the healing process?

We should not see ourselves as static or separate from each other. But this is part of the problem – we do! We may feel lonely and isolated or conversely, we may feel overwhelmed by other people and experience a desperate need to be on our own. However hard we try, though, we are an important part of a whole. Energy is intrinsic to our nature, even though we may not be directly aware of it.

Science is proving that healing – working with energy – is at the very least plausible and the concept of healing energy is gradually becoming more accepted. Through the use of Kirlian photography, a technique that reveals a subtle body or bioplasma around the body of all living things, we can actually see this energy.

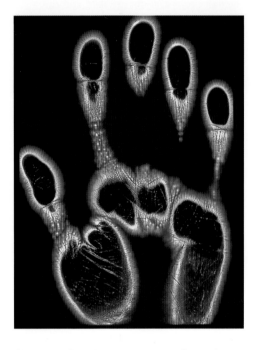

Kirlian photograph of a human hand: a photographic image is obtained due to the high energy interactions between the subject and an applied electrical field.

Photographs of energy outputs have also been taken during the healing process to show some of the changes that take place.

In truth, the word energy means many things to many people. We often use the word to describe stamina or vitality. We may use it to refer to an unexplained feeling, or to describe someone who has a certain charisma. Our ability to define it is limited by experience and by the fact we are trying to describe the indescribable!

However, in this book we will be using the term 'energy' to refer to the energy that surrounds us and circulates through our bodies. In Eastern systems of faith and healing it is referred to as *prana* or *chi*. This describes the same energy a healer harnesses and works on to affect change.

energy fields

As individuals, we are each surrounded by our own personal energy fields, often known as the aura. We can all sense these fields, even though we may not be conscious of them, and some people can actually see them. They are able to see colours in the energy field and can diagnose distress or illness in others without touching them. The energies within these fields are constantly interacting – with each other, with the fields of other individuals and with the environment as a whole.

There are four fields (or layers) radiating out from a person in a curved, almost egg-shaped, fashion. The field which is closest to the body is known as the etheric or vital energy field. You can often feel it by holding your hand about one to 5 cm/2 inches away from your arm, or you can see it by half-closing your eyes as you look at another person. This field is closely connected to the physical body, and is the one we shall be using in healing massage.

The etheric field is composed of a complex structure of energy lines linked to every cell in the body. It is concerned with energy exchange and assimilation.

The next two fields, the emotional and mental, are often linked together and are known as the astral field. The emotional field extends up to 1¼ metre/4 feet around the body and is charged with our feelings and emotions. What we feel changes its patterns. The mental field is concerned with intellect and rational thinking and is influenced by emotions. Ideas and images are connected with this field and these can often be directed, or projected, over great distances.

The fourth field is known as the causal or spiritual field and is connected to the universal whole. From here comes wisdom, compassion and intuition.

These four fields are constantly changing and interacting. Imbalances may permeate our vital energy field and result in physical disease.

the aura

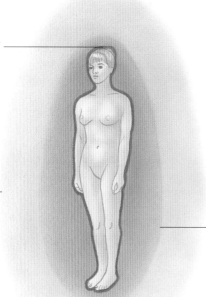

The etheric or vital energy field is closest to the physical body, radiating outward by approximately 5 cm/2 inches from the body.

The causal or spiritual field is connected to the universal whole and can extend outward to infinity.

The astral field comprises both the emotional field, which extends up to 1¼ metres/4 feet from the body, and the mental field, which can be directed or projected over great distances.

energy centres

the chakras

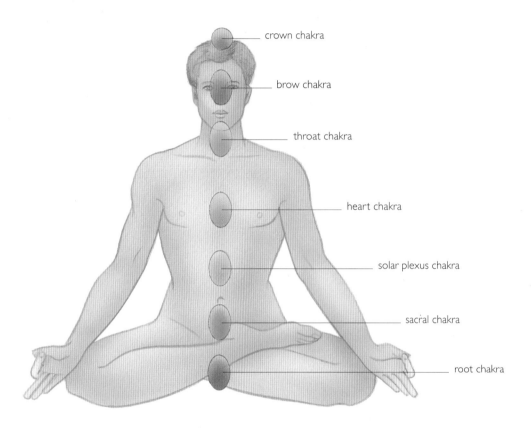

crown chakra

brow chakra

throat chakra

heart chakra

solar plexus chakra

sacral chakra

root chakra

Where concentrations of lines in the vital energy field cross, there are chakras. Chakra is a Sanskrit word which roughly translates as wheel. There are seven main chakras, or energy centres, associated with the body. They are described as spinning vortices and are concerned with the exchange of energies, both within the physical body and between the body and its subtle energy fields. Each of these main chakras is related to the nervous system and they are situated at the site of nerve ganglia or plexuses. They also relate to the endocrine system, again each chakra corresponding to, and interacting with, glands within the body.

The seven chakras are positioned the length of the spine and may be sensed at both the front and back of the body. They act rather like energy transformers, supplying the body with vital energy. The energy travels through pathways within the body where many other, smaller, energy centres are found. For example, there are secondary chakras in the hands. Each chakra is connected with a certain area of the body and has an effect on the organs within that area. In addition, each chakra is associated with a colour and certain emotional and psychological attributes. Many of the Eastern, and indeed Western, traditions have models for these human energy patterns. Each tradition often has a slightly different model, so it is easy for a certain degree of confusion to arise. Bear in mind that any

energy centres

the endocrine system

introduction

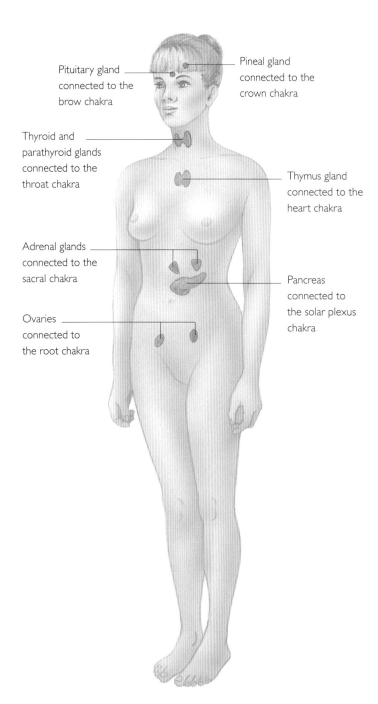

Pituitary gland connected to the brow chakra

Pineal gland connected to the crown chakra

Thyroid and parathyroid glands connected to the throat chakra

Thymus gland connected to the heart chakra

Adrenal glands connected to the sacral chakra

Pancreas connected to the solar plexus chakra

Ovaries connected to the root chakra

book you consult will say something different. However, these models are for information and reference only. As you delve deeper into the subject of healing and start to gain practical experience, you will find that your insight and under-standing will develop and grow.

The first chakra is known as the root or base chakra. It controls the gonads and ovaries. Its colour is red and it is associated with creative energy. It is located at the base of the spine and controls the reproductive system and the spinal column. This chakra connects us most strongly to the physical and is concerned with sexual, dynamic energy, survival and having our feet planted firmly on the ground. This chakra is our base or powerhouse, as it affects the balance of the other chakras.

The second chakra is located in the abdomen and controls the adrenal glands. It is associated with the pelvis, abdomen and lumbar spine but also controls the bladder, kidneys (often associated with fear) and the digestive process. This chakra is sometimes also linked to the spleen and is said to play an important part in the functioning of the immune system. Its colour is orange and it relates to vitality, sexuality and balance. It is very important in yoga and martial arts.

The third centre is located at the solar plexus. It controls the pancreas and is associated with the stomach, liver and spleen. Its colour is yellow and it is connected to the intellect and raw emotional energy. Emotional imbalances or an overflow of emotions – anger, for example, often show up here. This centre can be associated with the ego or the will. Those who feel stressed or who are psychically sensitive may feel tension in this area.

The heart chakra controls the thymus gland. This chakra is connected to the heart and circulation and the chest and lower lungs. This gland plays an important role in the immune system. Its colour is green and it is connected with love, compassion and feeling. In order to heal you need your heart, but beware: this centre easily becomes unbalanced or overloaded.

The next chakra is located in the throat and is connected to the thyroid gland. The associated organs are the lungs and respiratory system and the throat and upper thorax. Its colour is blue and it relates to our abilities of expression, communication and creativity. Any constriction in this area may result in, for example, sore throats or stiff shoulders. Blue is often associated with healing.

The sixth chakra is located in the brow and governs the pituitary gland. This is the centre often known as the 'third eye'. It is connected with the base of the skull and the *medulla oblongata*. Its colour is indigo and it is associated with wisdom, knowledge, intuition and insight. This chakra plays an important role in our healing potential and is also connected to psychic ability. It may, however, cause problems if too much energy is centred here before the rest of one's energies have developed and are in balance.

Finally, we come to the crown chakra, located at the crown of the head and connected to the pineal gland. This centre relates to the top of the head and the cerebral cortex. Its colour is violet and it is concerned with consciousness, creativity and the spiritual side of our nature. It also represents our highest aspirations and the potential we have to be connected to all things.

A cautionary word

We would all like to see ourselves as psychic or spiritual but concentrating on these aspects alone can lead to imbalance and disturbance. All our centres need to be balanced – and we must have a good solid base on all levels before we can begin to build upon them.

the human anatomy

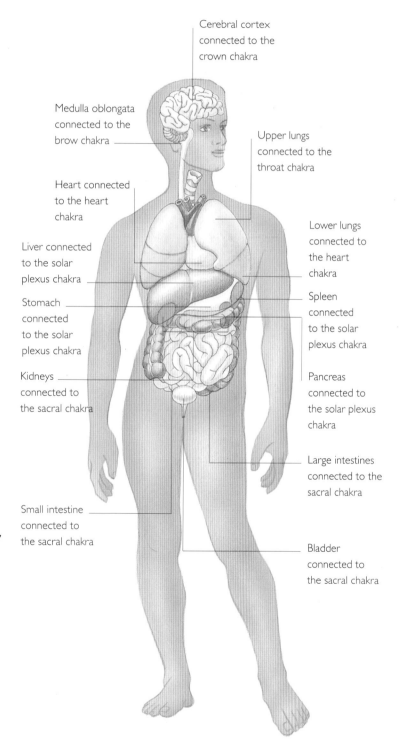

Cerebral cortex connected to the crown chakra

Medulla oblongata connected to the brow chakra

Upper lungs connected to the throat chakra

Heart connected to the heart chakra

Lower lungs connected to the heart chakra

Liver connected to the solar plexus chakra

Stomach connected to the solar plexus chakra

Spleen connected to the solar plexus chakra

Kidneys connected to the sacral chakra

Pancreas connected to the solar plexus chakra

Large intestines connected to the sacral chakra

Small intestine connected to the sacral chakra

Bladder connected to the sacral chakra

a short history

There is nothing new about the idea of healing. Throughout history all peoples, cultures, tribes and civilizations have held beliefs that mind, body and soul, health, sickness and the powers of healing are inextricably linked and bound together. For example, in the native cultures of Africa, Asia, North America and Australia, traditions of healing, together with a harmonious relationship and a respect for nature, are practised today as they were in ancient times.

Medicine men, healers, shamen and priests have always had a part to play in any culture or nation, looking after the spiritual and physical health of their particular society. In the Eastern civilizations of India, Tibet and China, the effect of the mind and spirit on the physical body and health has always been acknowledged and inter-woven within systems of practice and thought. Ancient healing practices are still being passed down today, while the healing powers of gurus and yogis remain legendary.

We can look back to ancient Egypt and Greece to find early examples of those who have influenced us. One of the earliest examples of a healer priest was Imhotep, born in ancient Egypt in the 27th century BC and exalted as a deity after his death.

In ancient Greece Asklepios was renowned as a powerful healer. Like Imhotep, he was revered as a god after his death and temples were erected to him. His emblem, the staff and serpent, remain the symbol of medicine today. Pythagoras, another Greek philosopher, was born in the 6th century BC. He was a physician and healer who believed in the existence of a healing energy. He also believed that health was rooted in the harmonious relationship between body and soul.

In the 5th century BC, Hippocrates, the most celebrated physician in antiquity, believed in the healing power of nature to restore health and harmony, advocating sensible living to prevent disease. The Hippocratic oath encompasses his principles and ethics of medicine and still has to be taken by Western doctors before they can perform their skills.

Jesus Christ, like Mohammed and Buddha, was one of the greatest healers the world has known. There are over forty references to healings in the New Testament. Of particular significance was, and is, the healing power of the spirit. There are also references to healings in the Old Testament. The Essenes, a Jewish sect living 1–2 centuries BC, believed that living in harmony could heal disease.

The early Christians were powerful healers. However, around the 2nd century AD, healing became the province of the church, ministered by priests through the laying on of hands and, later, unction or anointing of oil. By the late Middle Ages, healing practices within the Church were receding. Claims of having healing powers were considered heresy and punishable by death. At the end of the 18th century came the Age of Reason and the flowering and elevation of science. This resulted in a mechanistic world view, which today we are only just acknowledging as incomplete.

In recent times there has once again been an upsurge of interest in the spirit, the power of the mind, the holistic approach and healing. Why has it suddenly become popular? Partly, I believe, because, technically advanced and materially advantaged as we are, there is something missing from most people's lives. Doctors' surgeries are filled with people suffering the modern disease of stress.

Very many of us now want a greater, more meaningful world view; we want to feel able to take responsibility for our own health. This is where healing plays an important part. Healing offers hope. This is something we can do for ourselves. Medical diagnoses may sometimes be so final that many people lose all heart. If disease itself cannot be cured, a change in our attitude or perspective can, at the very least, bring relief and greater peace of mind.

introduction

Crowds of the sick and ailing gather to be healed by Hesso von Reinach, renowned physician, German illuminated manuscript (1234–1276).

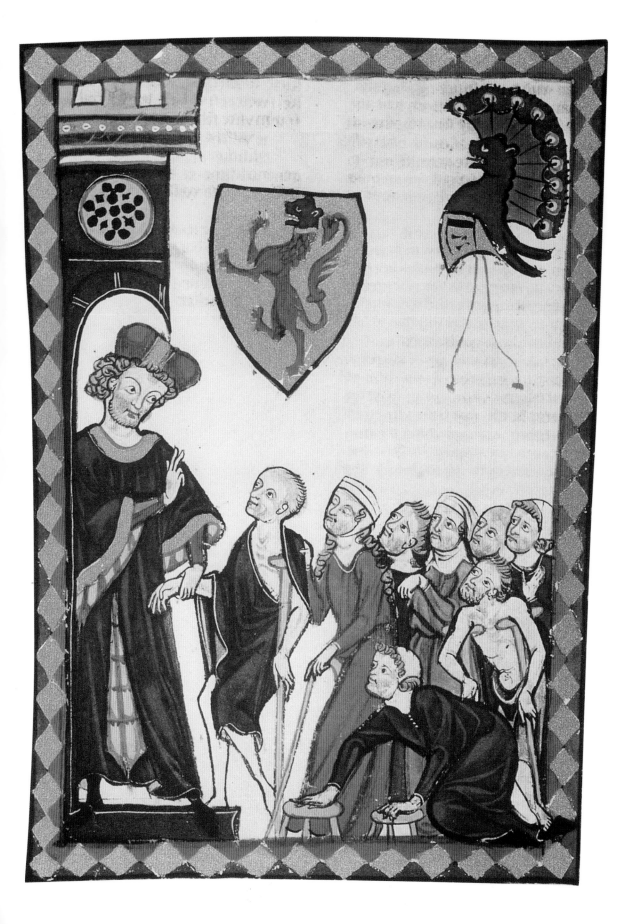

what makes a healer?

It is not the healer who is important, it is the healing itself. Healing is something that flows through you. Although energy can be directed, what is also provided is a structure within which healing can take place, prompting a replenishment of energies and a return to health. Openness, willingness and compassion are of prime importance, as are ability, self-discipline and an eagerness to learn. You also need to be practical. The greatest healers I have known have all had their feet planted firmly on the ground.

Healing involves self-knowledge and personal development, strength and a desire to do what is best. Many people develop healing and/or psychic abilities on their path of spiritual development. However, a fascination in phenomena does not help others, and that is what healing is all about.

Serious illness can bring about panic and fear. Often the healer's most important role is that of providing a positive attitude. Long illness can take its toll, and negativity creeps in. We would all like to be able to make everything all right but the trick is having the confidence of knowing that your efforts will achieve the best results for each person.

Can anybody heal? There are those who, as in any field, have special talents. For the rest of us, however, I believe we can achieve much through dedication and patience. At the least, what we can all do is begin to try.

Massage is a form of healing, of enabling the body to help itself. In the previous pages we have discussed various aspects of healing, but we are now going to do nothing so grand! We are simply going to incorporate a further dimension and explore ways of working with sensitivity to heighten massage.

Massage is a physical process so we are going to combine these skills with healing techniques which involve a high degree of touch. The gentle aspect of healing massage is especially helpful for those who are ill or in need of care. In a healing massage we will work at treating the whole person and attend to common problems without trying to cure any particular disease. A healing massage will help a person to relax and regain their sense of balance. This is the best starting point from which healing can then take place.

introduction

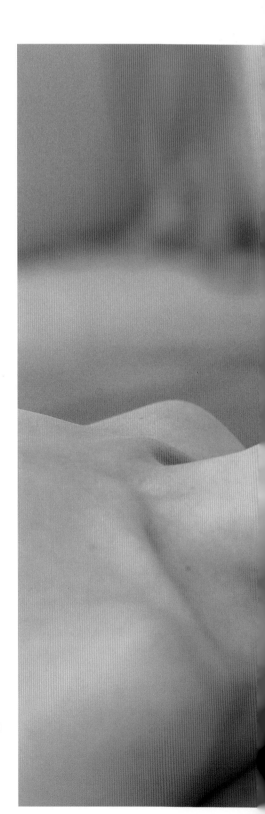

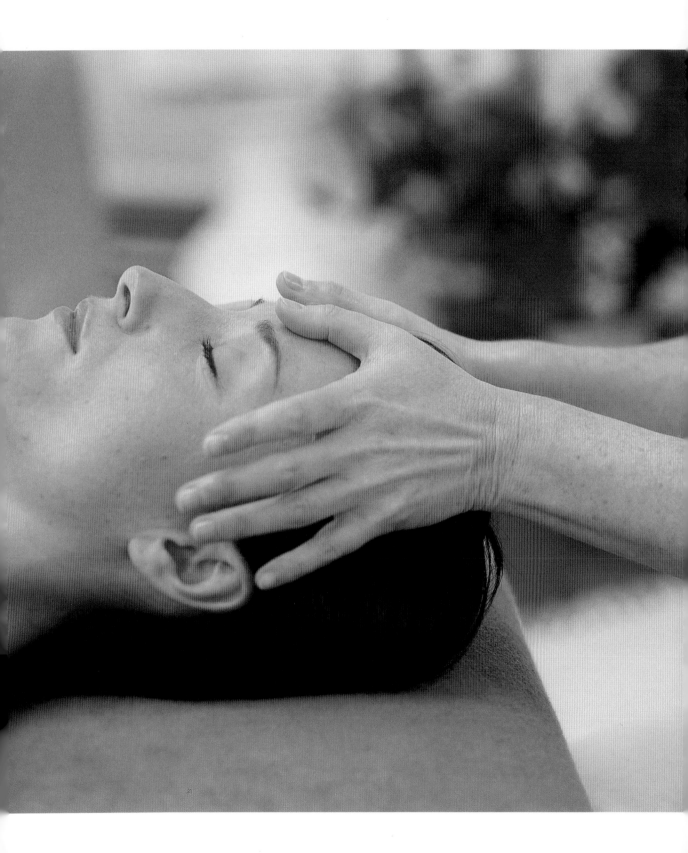

healing techniques

Healing is a learning experience. If you are a novice to healing massage you should try not to become anxious about your technique – it can only improve with practice. Have confidence that your partner will get what they need from the massage and do the best you are able to do. The most rewarding results usually come from letting things happen naturally, rather than trying to predict an outcome. As you practise the techniques, pay attention to the sensations you feel, even if they seem unimportant. This way you build up a holistic experience of what healing massage is about – which is as much about you and your feelings as it is about your partner's.

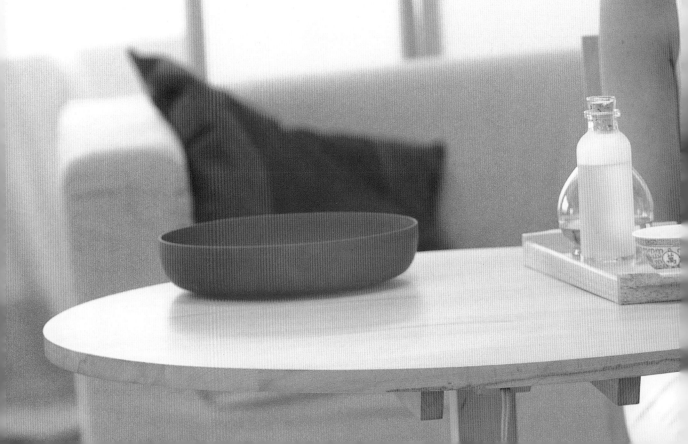

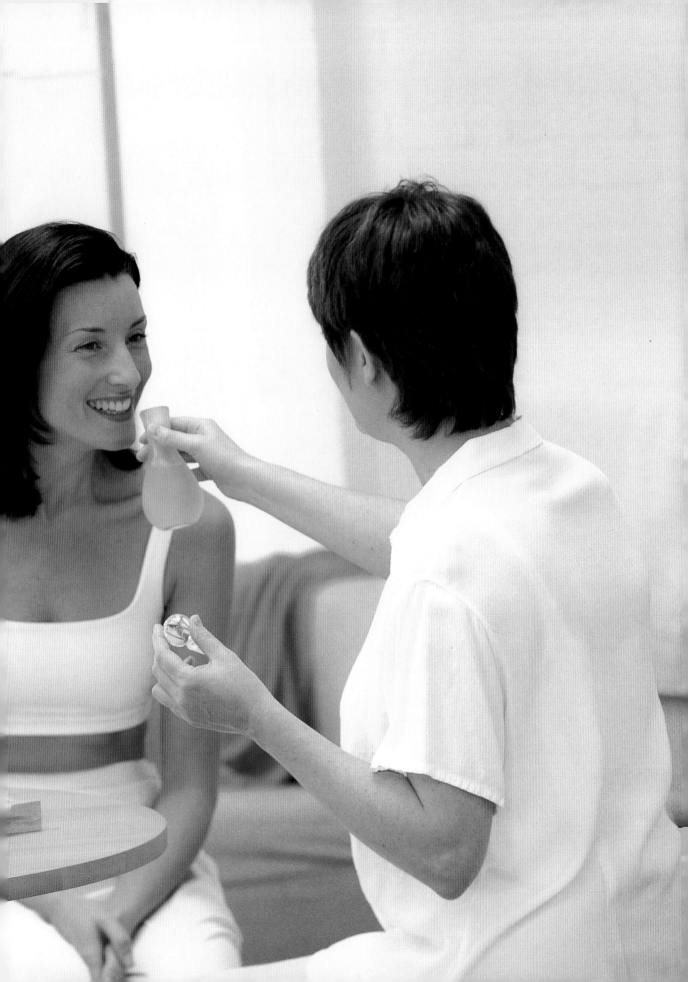

rubbing hands

Before experimenting with any of the other techniques, try this simple exercise to get a sense of what energy feels like. It is important to feel your way around. Although instructions are necessary to point you in the right direction, it is your own sense of discovery and development that will give you confidence. This exercise is for anyone. Concentrate on the feeling in your hands as they move together and apart. Make a note of any particular sensations you experience, such as warmth, cold or tingling. Do not think about it, simply focus on what you feel.

Step 1

Stand or sit in a relaxed position and breathe naturally. Begin rubbing your hands together quite vigorously, as if trying to keep warm. Rub until you feel heat in your palms, then slowly draw your hands apart. You may find they spring open quite naturally.

Step 2

When your hands are about a shoulder-width apart, stop and slowly bring them back towards each other again. Keep relaxed, with your palms rounded and facing each other. At a certain point – which differs for each person but is roughly 12–20 cm/5–8 inches apart – you will feel a slight springiness between your hands, like two magnets coming together.

Step 3

Now experiment by drawing your hands further apart and then bringing them towards each other, without losing the sensation between them. Keep your arms and hands relaxed, as if you were holding a delicate ball. The distinctive sensation is the energy between your hands.

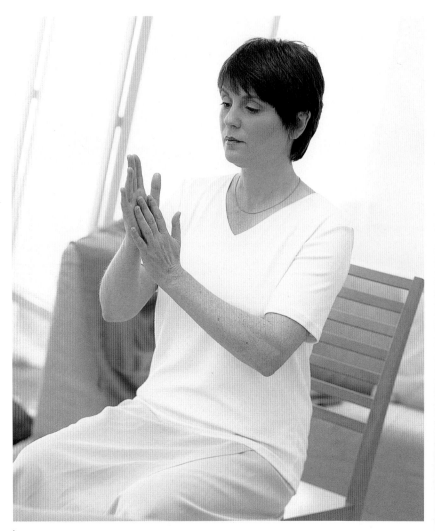

1

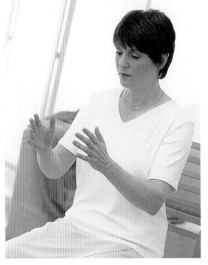

2

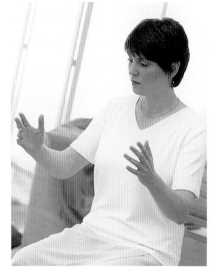

3

sensing

Now you have got a sense of what energy feels like, the next step is to get a sense of another person. Make sure it is someone who is sympathetic to what you are doing, as this will help to build your confidence. You may find you can pick up a lot of information through your hands. Keep an open mind towards the sensations you feel and maintain a general awareness, rather than thinking about it. Remember, healing is not an analytical process and is helped by relaxation rather than mental effort.

Step 1

This exercise may be done standing or sitting. Make sure you are comfortable and relaxed, with your feet a shoulder-width apart and planted firmly on the ground. Now, gently bring one hand up towards your partner's back. As you move your hand slowly towards your partner, be aware of the sensations you feel. Stop roughly 5–7 cm/2–3 inches away from your partner.

Step 2

As in the previous exercise, slowly draw your hand away, then bring it back towards your partner without actually touching their back. Note the sensations you feel in your hand, as well as anything else about your partner that becomes apparent. Try this several times. When you finish, stroke down to your partner's lower back, making sure you do not move away abruptly.

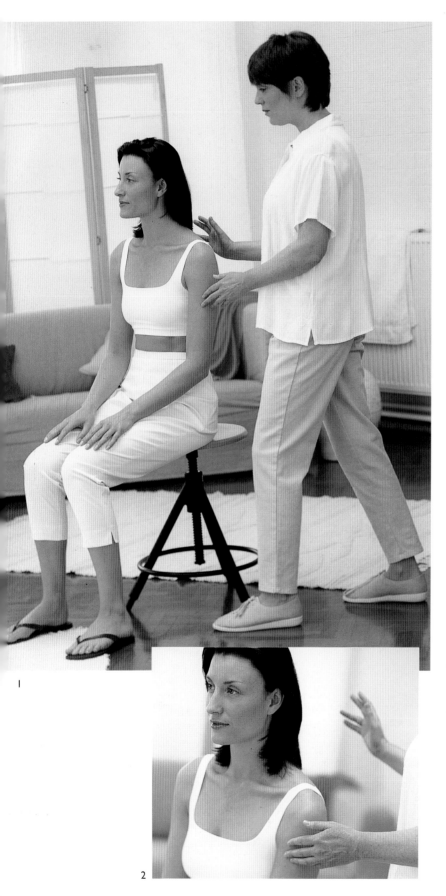

1

2

posture

As the giver or healer, the way you hold yourself is of great importance. Your body and hands are your tools. If you are not positioned correctly, and feeling relaxed and comfortable, the information you receive may be impaired and you will be less able to move freely. Working with massage as well as healing can easily put a strain on the body and tire you more quickly. Make sure your spine is straight when you work and bend from the legs and hips. Relax your shoulders and round out your upper back and arms so that you have space to perform the movements. Make sure you are well balanced, and you feel your feet in contact with the ground. When you are comfortable your mind can relax, and your partner will feel able to relax too.

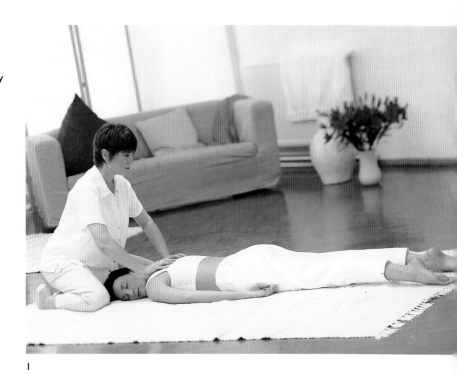

1

Step 1

It is perfectly possible, and indeed a lot more intimate, to give your massage on the floor. Follow the rules of keeping your spine straight while kneeling or sitting back on your heels. Begin the massage by centring yourself, then leaning your whole body forwards to begin the strokes. Kneeling on cushions or padding makes it easier on your knees.

Step 2

Working on the floor can be more physical than standing at a table as it enables you to put your whole body into the strokes. Move from the hips to avoid rounding your shoulders and, when you need extra support, change position so that your lower body rather than the upper part takes your partner's weight.

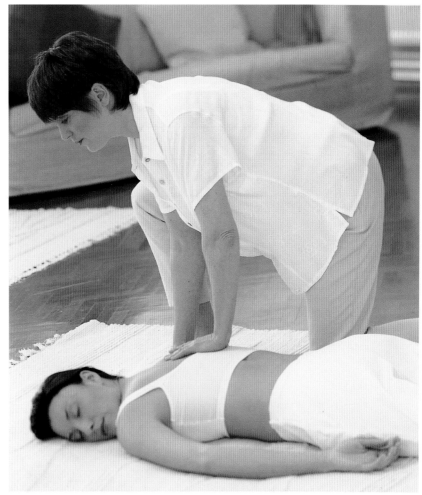

2

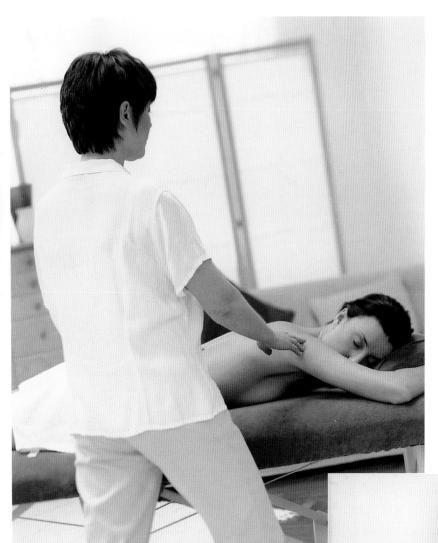

Step 3

The advantage of using a table is that it is easier on your back and more suitable if you are giving a lot of massage. However, you need to make sure it is the right height for you so you can work effectively. Stand square on to the table with your feet firmly on the ground, but move one leg behind the other for movements that would otherwise involve a twist. Bend from the knees and hips.

Step 4

A stool can be invaluable when working on your partner's face or feet. It allows you to maintain a comfortable, steady position and avoid leaning too far over your partner. Strangely enough, there is a constant pull towards the massage surface. Try to avoid giving in to this as it is not only bad for your posture, but it can also feel intrusive to the other person.

3

4

giving

Now that we have experimented with sensing our own energy and that of our partner, we are going to sense specific areas of our partner's body and then send some energy to them through our hands. This is not as difficult as it sounds. The key, as always, is to stay relaxed and not try to force anything. Imagine that energy is travelling through your hands – even if you don't yet feel it – and you will find it will come eventually. Healing should feel natural and easy. If you feel dramatic effects, the chances are you are trying too hard and feeling your own or your partner's resistance.

Step 1

Your partner should lie face down and be as relaxed as possible. Stand square to your partner, shoulders relaxed and feet firmly on the ground. Slowly bring your hands up over your partner's back, roughly 5–15 cm/2–6 inches away from their body. Have one hand positioned above their shoulder blades with the other above the lower back.

Step 2

Slowly lower both hands on to your partner's back, noting any sensations as you do so. Rest your hands on your partner's body, without exerting any pressure, and imagine energy coming out through your hands. There is no need to direct this energy to any particular place, just imagine it flowing through your hands.

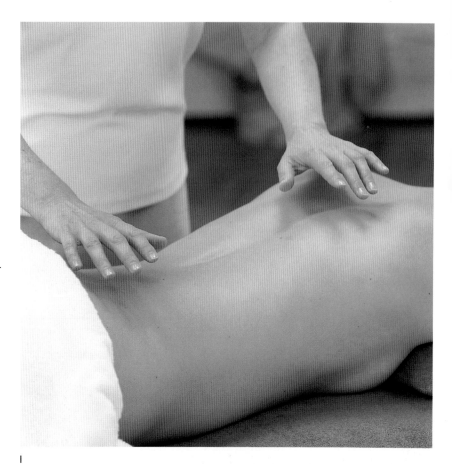

1

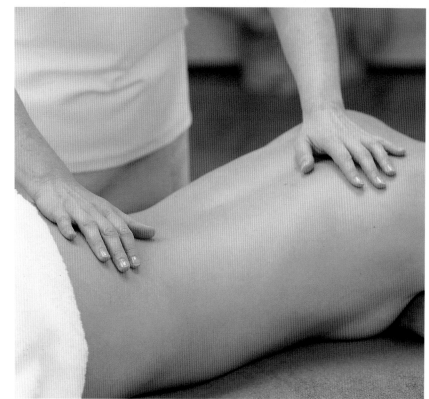

2

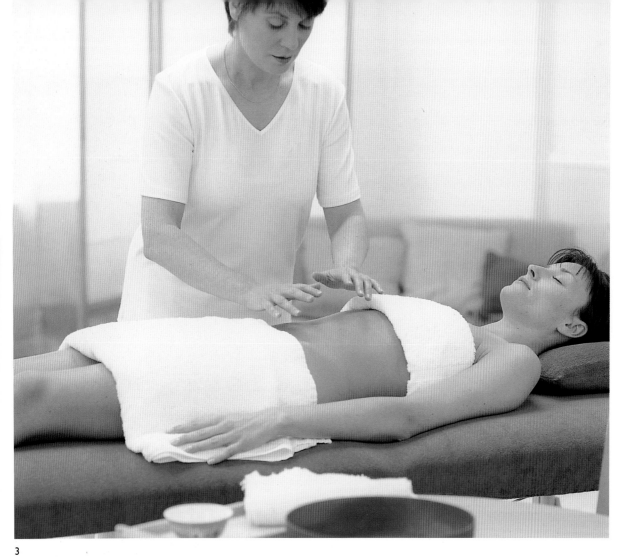

3

Step 3

Your partner lies on their back. Stand square to your partner, as before, and hold your hands over your partner's abdomen, 5 cm/2 inches away. Keep your hands there for a few moments while you relax your mind and note any sensations you feel. Remember, the front of the body is vulnerable so perform each step with sensitivity.

Step 4

Slowly lower your hands, so one is resting just below the solar plexus and the other is below the navel. Once more imagine energy travelling from your body and out through your hands. Check how this feels for your partner. Always make sure you are giving, not taking, and don't try too hard to get a 'result'.

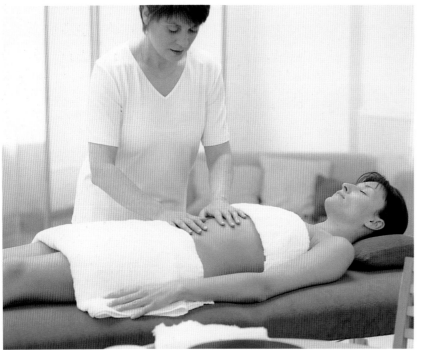

4

connecting

It may seem strange but many people do not feel themselves as physically 'whole'. They may be aware of certain parts of their body but not others, typically the lower body and legs. This technique helps to connect different areas of the body to others, using a very light touch.

Step 1

Rest your hands on the areas you wish to connect, without resting your weight on your partner. One hand may feel as if it is full while the other may feel empty. Imagine your partner's energy flowing from one area to the other.

Step 2

Place one hand over your partner's lower back, the other over the sole of the foot. Be aware of the sensations in your hands and how these parts of the body feel. Your partner's feet may feel cold. Now imagine energy running from the lower back to the foot. When you notice a change in sensation, or after fifteen seconds, repeat on the other leg.

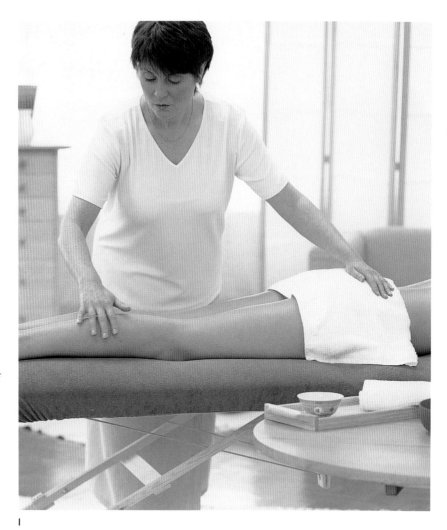

1

healing techniques

2

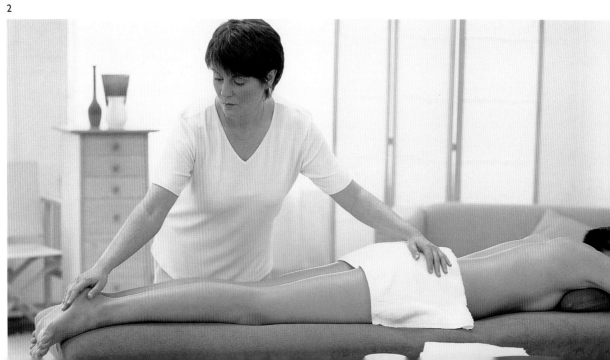

circling

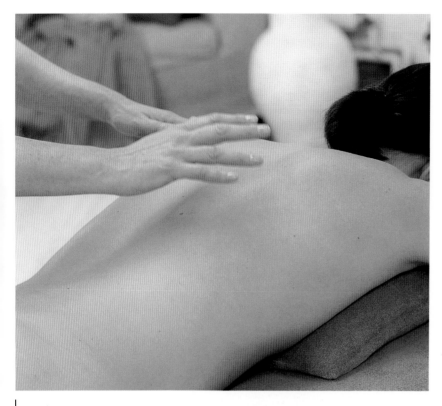

1

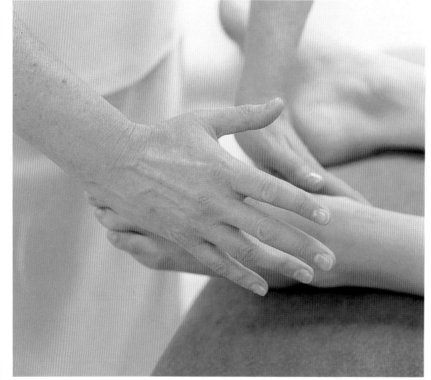

2

Sometimes you may notice that your partner feels tense or weak in a certain area, or there may be some injury where you cannot actually touch the body. Gently circling your hand, without touching, above the affected area can help to bring relief. Hold your hand roughly 6 cm/3 inches away from the body and then relax, without trying to influence what happens. Strangely enough, trying can reduce the effect. The movements should be anticlockwise over the back of the body but clockwise over the front. Avoid the face and chest. You will get a feel about how long to do this, but generally, you should not do this for more than 30 seconds.

Step 1

Bring your hand to roughly 5–15 cm/2–6 inches above your partner's upper back, over the area between the shoulder blades. Notice any sensations in your hand or any feeling you get about your partner before you start. Gently circle your hand anticlockwise over the area, then bring it to rest on the back.

Step 2

Place your hand 5 cm/2 inches away from your partner's ankle, then begin small circles away from the body. Draw your hand further away and circle again, noting any sensations you feel. Check how this is affecting your partner and then gently bring your hand to rest over the foot.

balancing

Balancing your partner is usually done at the end of any specific work you have been doing. More often than not our energy tends to be held in the upper body, upper back and chest, rather than being balanced and centred. Holding your hands over your partner helps them to relax and encourages awareness downwards, through the body. Balancing can be done on both back and front, but once again, do not work on the head, face or chest. Breathe into your hands as you rest there, without leaning on your partner, and believe that you are feeling relaxed and positive. Note any warmth or tingling in your hands.

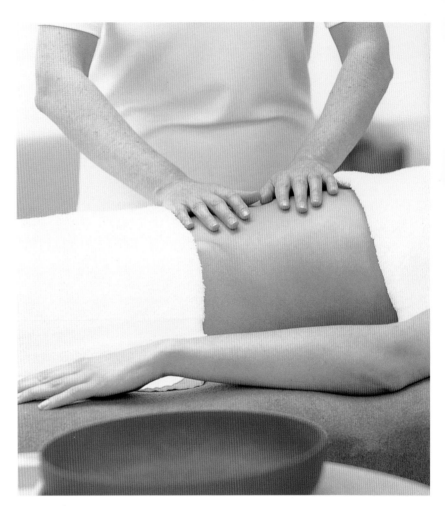

Step 1

Stand in a relaxed position, square to your partner. Now place your hands over the abdomen, one hand just below the solar plexus, the other just below the navel. Make sure your arms, hands and mind are relaxed. Breathe in time with your partner and let your hands rise and fall with their breath. Do not press or try to control in any way.

releasing

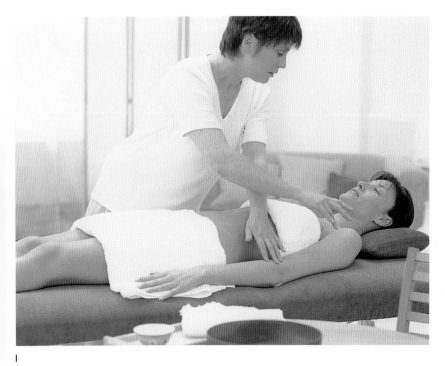

This technique is particularly useful after you have been working on specific areas of the body. As physical tension releases, or if one area feels overactive, you can draw nervous tension from the upper or lower body downwards, through the arms and legs. These movements are relatively quick, light and barely touch the body. You can cover the entire limb or begin the movements just above the hands or feet. As you move your hands, imagine that energy is coming down your partner's limbs and being released through the fingers or toes. This will help to release tension and at the same time energize your partner.

Step 1

Stand at the lower part of your partner's body. Starting at the top of the shoulder, sweep your hands lightly over and right the way down the arm in a succession of small movements. Imagine any nervous energy moving with your hands and releasing out through the fingers. Repeat this several times, then move to the other side and repeat on the opposite arm.

Step 2

Stand at the lower part of your partner's body. Once more, begin the small sweeping movements over the hip and ripple down the leg, imagining energy releasing through the toes. Change position and repeat on the other leg. Relax and then rest both hands gently over the feet.

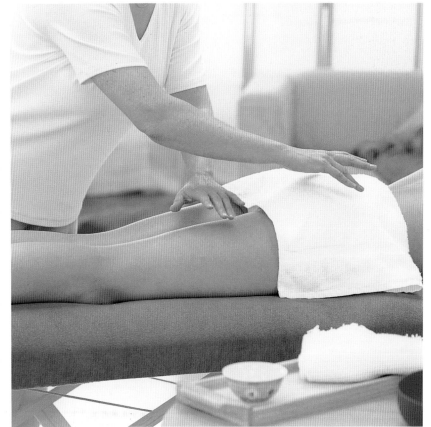

1

2

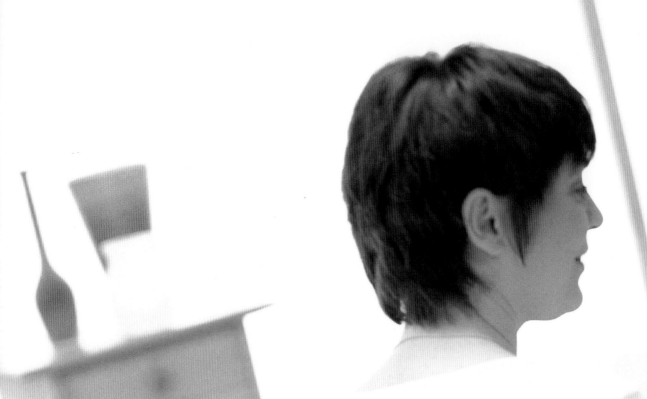

massage techniques

Although healing massage is similar to other forms of massage, what makes it different is the way you use the techniques and the reasons for applying them. As with the techniques in the healing section, massage techniques need to be practised with a partner. Note the sensations you both experience, so that you can use the information later. Your body, and particularly your hands, are your best allies and need to be used and treated with sensitivity. Massage teaches you about your partner's physical patterns and areas of muscular tension, giving you an important insight into what techniques may be beneficial. It also increases receptivity and encourages healing.

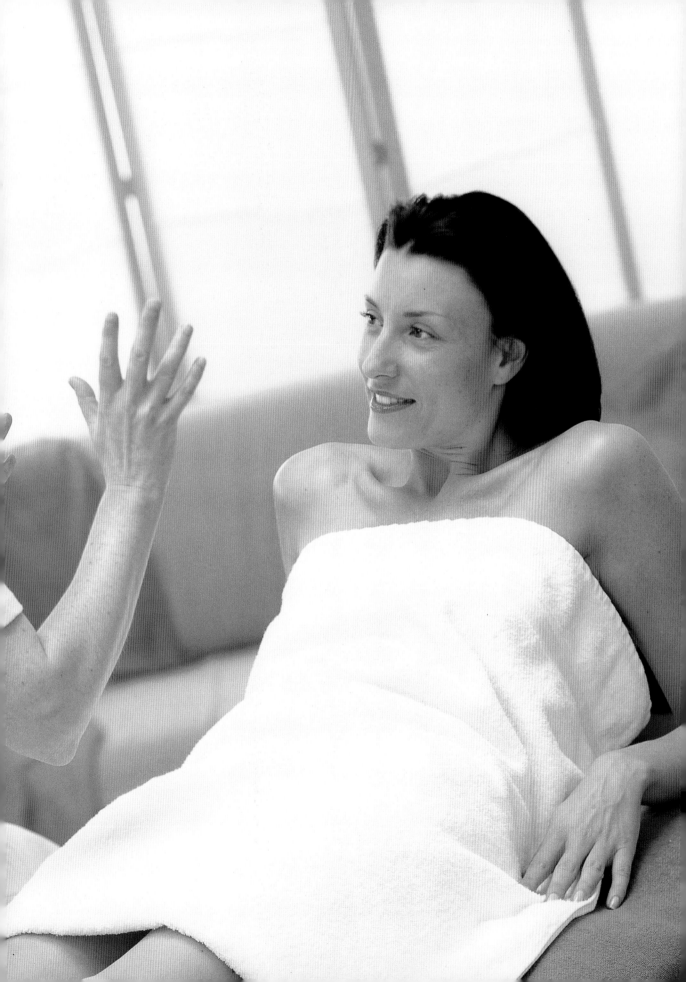

breathing

What makes healing massage different is the sensitivity involved, the focus on the use of energy and the link with healing techniques through the hands. The use of the breath to focus awareness and energize your hands is the first – but very important – step which takes place before physical contact. By standing at your partner's head, they can relax while you take a few moments to centre yourself and breathe into your hands. This is also a moment to focus on the purpose of the massage, and to dedicate it if you wish to. This takes place only once, but will set the tone of the massage. It also acts as a boundary: from here, your sensitivities will be heightened until you finish the massage.

Step 1

Stand, or kneel, at the head of your partner, a 5 cm/2 inches away from the surface you are working on. Relax, so that your body is balanced and your feet are firmly on the ground. Imagine your energy running through your legs, through your feet and into the ground. When you are ready, breathe in a relaxed way through your abdomen. Breathe in once again, and as you breathe out, imagine the energy moving down your arms and into your hands.

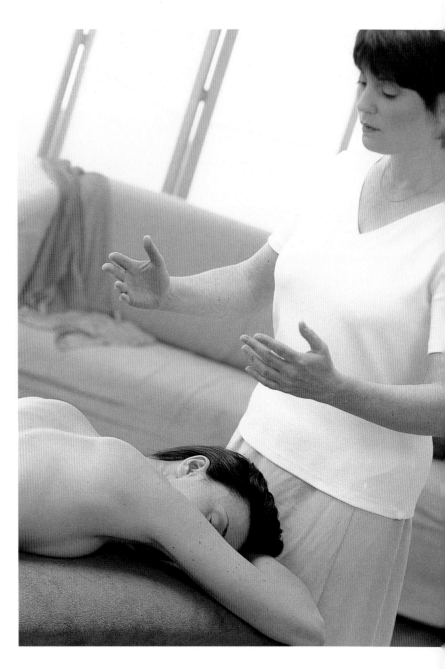

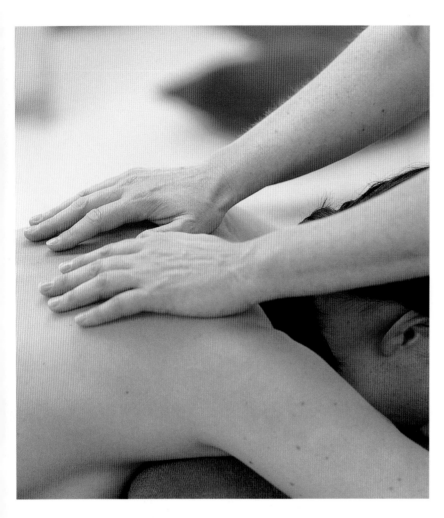

contact

This first physical contact between you and your partner follows on naturally from the previous step, and marks the beginning of the massage. Once your hands feel alive and energized, place them gently but firmly on your partner's back. This touch is important. You will already have picked up many clues about your partner from the way they sit, talk and feel. This is where you join together and provides an opportunity for your hands to pick up information. Notice what you feel. Your partner will also get a physical sense of you and will be reassured by the quality of your touch. Remember that healing is taking place within the framework of the massage, and as massage is a physical skill, you need to be centred and focused on touch.

Step 1

From the same position, place your hands gently on your partner's upper back. Rest your hands, without leaning or applying pressure. Make sure you are giving and your attention is directed towards your partner. Note any sensations in your hands, and any clues you get, such as the feel and temperature of your partner's skin, any tension or relaxation, and whether or not they are receptive.

stroking

We now come to the first of the actual massage techniques. Stroking is one of the gentle, light pressure techniques. It is usually performed at the end of a particular massage sequence focused on a specific area of the body. Stroking is pleasurable and connects sensations in the area that has just been massaged. It draws attention to that part of the body and relaxes, revitalizes and stimulates the skin. When performed slowly it has a calming, soothing effect. Use the tips of your fingers along the length of the back or limb so that you produce a rhythmic, rippling sensation.

1 Back

Stand facing up your partner's body. Reach to the upper back and then stroke down its length with your fingertips. It is more effective to use several small strokes so you get a wave-like effect. Repeat this several times, imagining you are connecting the upper and lower back.

2 Legs

Stand at your partner's feet and work on the back of the leg, reaching up to the thigh and stroking downwards towards the ankle. Continue the movement over the feet and toes. Keep your strokes to the centre of the leg and imagine you are relaxing and connecting the whole leg, from hip to toe.

3 Feet

Stroke your partner's feet to relax or energize them. Stroke over the ankle, down the foot and over the toes, imagining your partner's energy flowing to the toes. Sometimes holding the foot with one hand feels reassuring. You can then just stroke with your other hand.

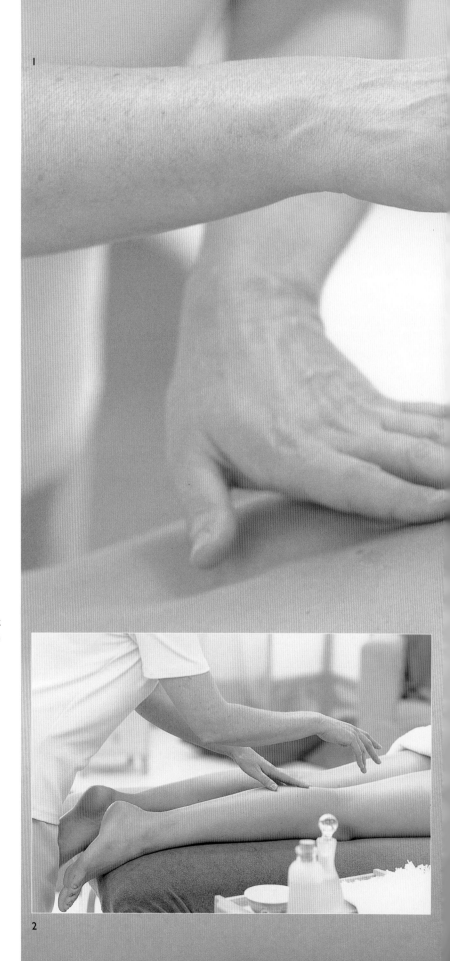

1

2

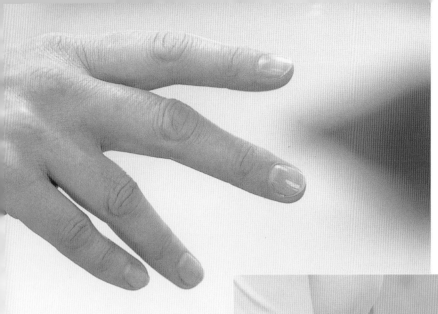

4 Hands

After working on the arm or shoulder, finish the sequence by stroking right from the shoulder down over the arm and wrist to the fingertips. Keeping your wrists relaxed, stroke in a series of waves, bringing your partner's attention down to the fingers.

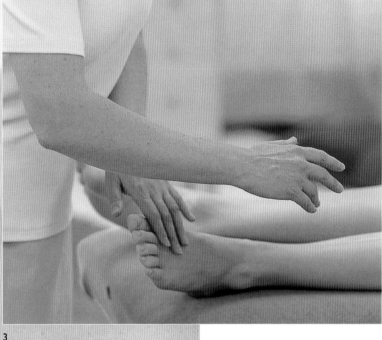

3

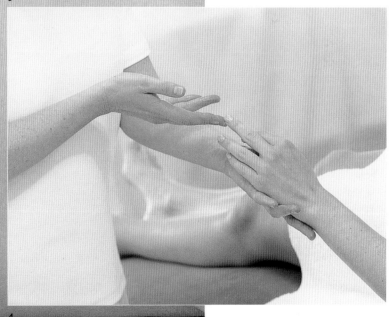

4

rocking

Rocking is another light pressure stroke. People sometimes find it difficult to relax, even if they want to. Both the muscles and joints can become stiff with tension. Rocking the body or limbs is lighthearted, relaxing and effective, encouraging the body to loosen, let go, and return to a more natural movement. Rocking should be done using light pressure from the hands alternately, so that the result is a gentle, swaying effect. Move your hands up and down the area you are working on so that the whole limb is affected. The movements can be done early in the massage to help your partner relax, or after you have worked on a particular area of the body. Keep your arms and hands relaxed and let your own body move as you work.

1 Arms

Stand facing up your partner's body. Cup both hands on either side of the upper arm, starting as high as possible. Rock the arm back and forth between your hands, moving down towards the wrist. It may help to actually lift the arm and get your hands underneath. You can work quite quickly on the wrist, and then stroke over the fingers.

2 Legs

Stand at your partner's feet. Place one hand on the outside and the other on the inside of the thigh, keeping well clear of the groin. Gently rock the leg between your hands, imagining you are releasing all tension around the joints. Move your position as you work towards the ankle, so that your partner experiences one smooth movement. End by stroking over the toes.

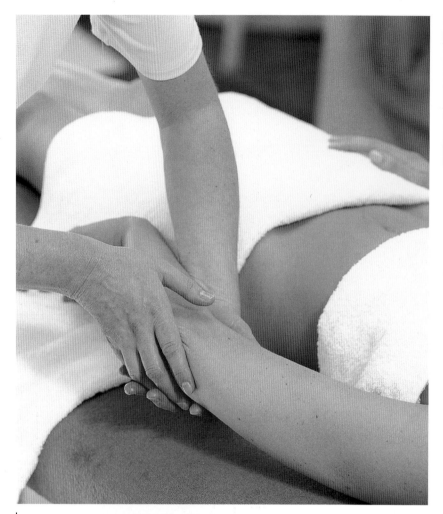

1

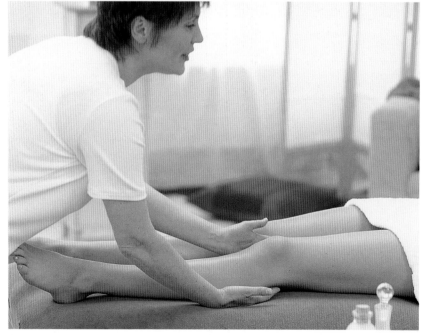

2

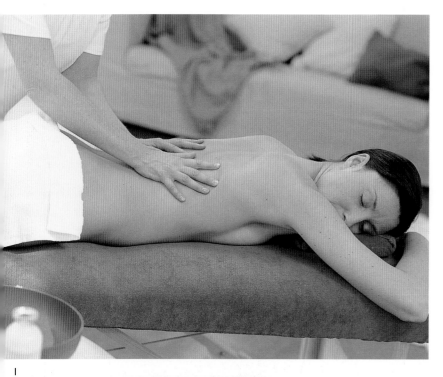

1

effleurage

This is the last of the light pressure strokes. Effleurage is a gentle, fan-like stroke used at the beginning of any sequence where you are using oil. It serves to spread the oil over the skin, relaxes the surface of the muscles and also tells you a great deal about your partner's state of health. You may also get an impression of any strong emotions. Mentally note anything you feel. As you work, imagine your strokes relaxing your partner and releasing built-up tension from the muscles. Effleurage uses the flat of the hand, with fingers and wrists relaxed so the movements feel smooth and rhythmic.

1 Back

Rub a little oil between your hands and position yourself at your partner's lower back, facing up the body. Gently place your hands side by side over the lower back and then glide slowly up towards the neck. As you reach the shoulders, let your hands fan out to the sides and then come lightly down the sides of the body. Repeat several times.

2 Chest

Stand at your partner's head. Rub a little oil between your hands and place your fingertips at the top of the chest. Glide down the centre, keeping away from the breasts. Let your hands fan out around the bottom of the ribcage and then draw them back together to the top of the chest. Repeat the movement.

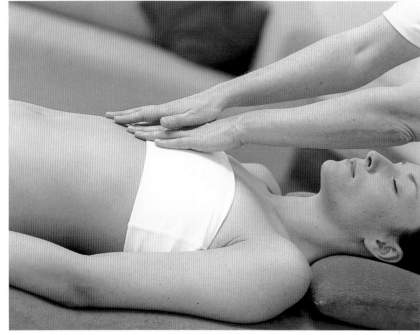

2

sweeping

Sweeping is a light to medium pressure stroke using the flat of the hand. It is used after squeezing the muscles, to relax them and to get a sense of stretching and opening out, both across and up the back. The muscles that run to the sides of the spine can become tight and contracted, resulting in a general stiffness and lack of movement. Working in a quick succession of strokes and applying pressure away from the spine helps to ease the muscles and encourage flexibility in the back. As you work, imagine you are easing pressure away from the spine, relaxing your own back and hands as you do so.

1 Back

Stand diagonally to your partner. Lightly place one hand on the muscles to the far side of the spine of your partner's lower back. Sweep your hand away from you and towards the side of the body. Repeat the stroke with your other hand slightly further up the back, continuing up to the shoulders. Repeat the whole sequence.

2 Hips

Stand square to your partner. Place one hand to the far side of the lower back, sweep round the hip and back towards you over the buttock. Repeat with the other hand. Imagine you are helping to stretch out the lower back. Apply pressure away from you, then ease it as your hands return.

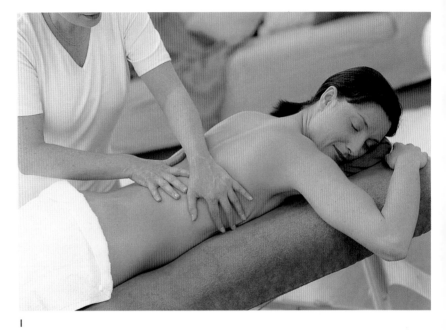

I

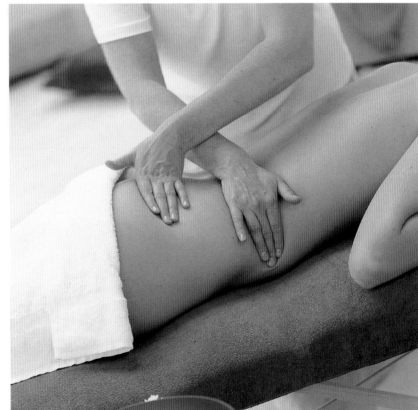

2

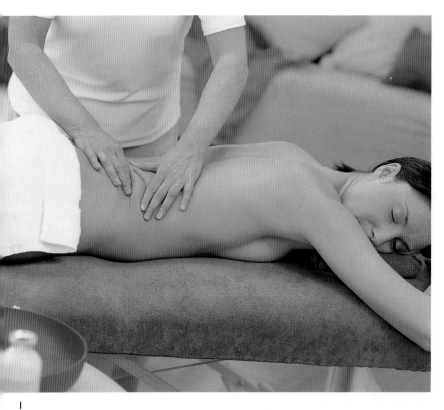

kneading

Kneading is a stroke requiring medium pressure. It is used after the muscles have been relaxed and some oil has been spread over the skin. Tension in the muscles constricts the flow of energy through the body. These movements, which are a little bit like kneading dough, work more deeply, to relax the muscles, release general tension and increase the circulation. Using thumb and fingers, the hands work alternately, pressing and squeezing the muscles in a rolling movement. Kneading is generally used over large, fleshy areas where the hands have ample room to work.

1 Back

Stand square to your partner's lower back, making sure you can lean across comfortably. First press into the band of muscle to the far side of the spine with one thumb and then roll back towards you with your fingers. Do the same with the other hand so that you are making a continuous, rhythmic movement. Work upwards to the shoulder.

2 Buttocks

Stand square to your partner. Once more, lean across and press into the opposite buttock with your thumb, rolling back towards you with your fingers. Repeat the movement over the fleshy areas. Make sure that the pressure is comfortable for your partner, and imagine that you are releasing tension around the lower back and hips.

1

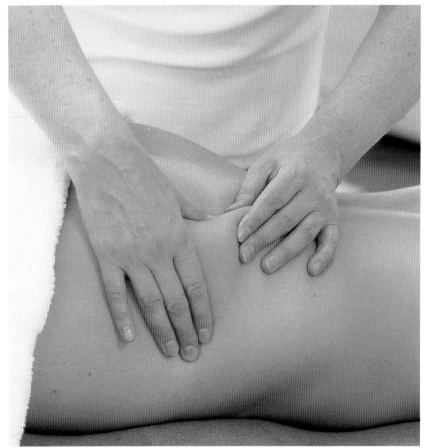

2

thumb spreading

Thumb spreading is a medium pressure stroke which uses the thumbs to apply pressure outwards over the muscles. The stroke covers one small area at a time, such as the sole of the foot or back of the knee. Spreading encourages the release of tension in the muscles or joints. Cupping the area you are working on with your hands provides a support for your partner and allows you to apply pressure with your thumbs. When you are working around the joints, remember to keep the pressure to a minimum.

1 Foot

Stand at your partner's feet. Lift the foot slightly, cupping it in your hands. Place your thumbs together over the sole of the foot, and gradually slide them apart, applying pressure as you do so. Squeeze the foot at the end of the movement. Repeat several times.

2 Knee

Stand facing up your partner's body. Cup your hands around the knee, without applying any pressure. Place your thumbs together at the back of the knee and then gently slide them outwards. Make sure your pressure is light and the movement is smooth. Imagine you are releasing tension around the joint and encouraging relaxation in the leg.

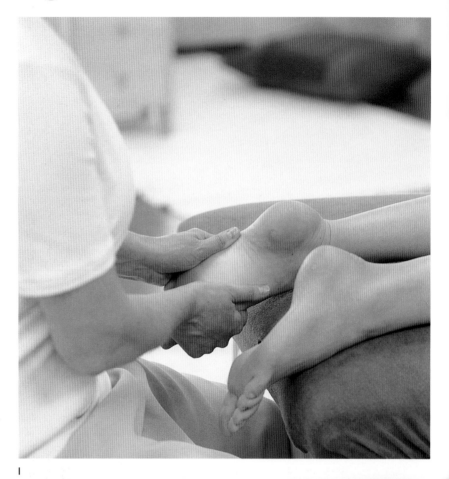

1

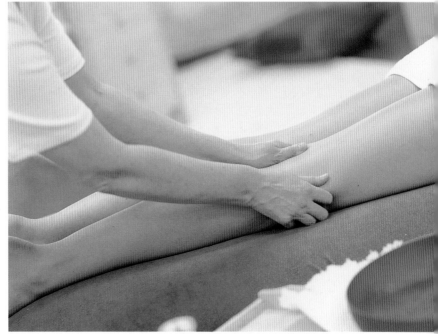

2

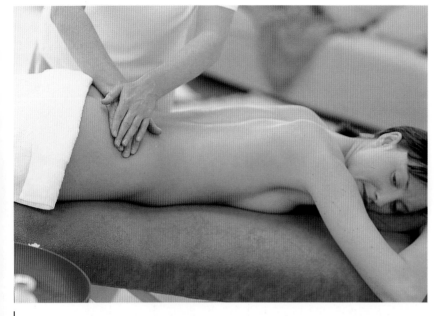

circling

Circling is a medium pressure stroke which uses the flat of the hand to circle over a fairly large area, usually the back and abdomen. Circling can be a relaxing, comforting stroke and is extremely helpful if your partner is upset, as it helps to sedate, soothe and diffuse nervous tension and emotion. Keep your hands relaxed and follow the body's contours. As with working away from the body, perform the movements in an anticlockwise direction over the back, and in a clockwise direction on the front. This is in line with the body's energy. The physical strokes can be followed by working 5 cm/2 inches away from the body.

1 Sacrum

Stand square to your partner. Place one hand over the sacrum (the bony triangle at the base of the spine) and the other hand lightly on top. Make fairly wide circles over the sacrum and lower back, using your upper hand for more pressure. Imagine you are relaxing and releasing the whole lower back area. Always check that the stroke feels comfortable.

2 Abdomen

Stand square to your partner. Begin circling over the abdomen with one hand, then follow the circle with the other. Always keep one hand in continuous contact with the body, lifting the other hand as they cross over. Never use too much pressure in this area and keep the movements slow, relaxing and smooth.

massage techniques

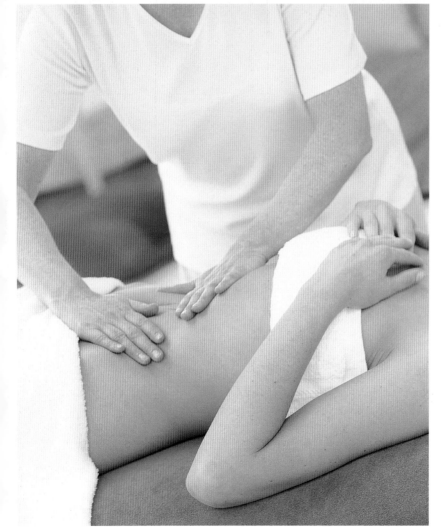

clearing (hands and feet)

This is a particular way of clearing tension and increasing relaxation in the hands and feet. It is a medium pressure stroke, and although it is not actually pinching, it looks that way as you draw down between the tendons. Energy centres are located in the hands and feet, which have a lot of work to do. However, when the muscles become tight they cannot function properly. These strokes help to relax both palms and soles. If your partner is having a problem with physical expression, it is beneficial to work on the hands and feet. Imagine you are helping to stimulate the blood flow.

1 Hands

Sit or stand facing your partner's body while supporting the hand. Reach up as high as you can between their first finger and thumb with your own thumb. Now, draw down between the bones towards the fingers, applying pressure underneath at the same time with your first finger. Repeat the movement between the bones across the hand.

2 Feet

Sit or stand at your partner's feet. Support the foot with one hand and place the thumb of your other hand as high up the foot as possible, between the big and second toes. Apply pressure with your middle finger underneath and draw back towards you, being careful to slide rather than dig inwards. Work your way across the foot.

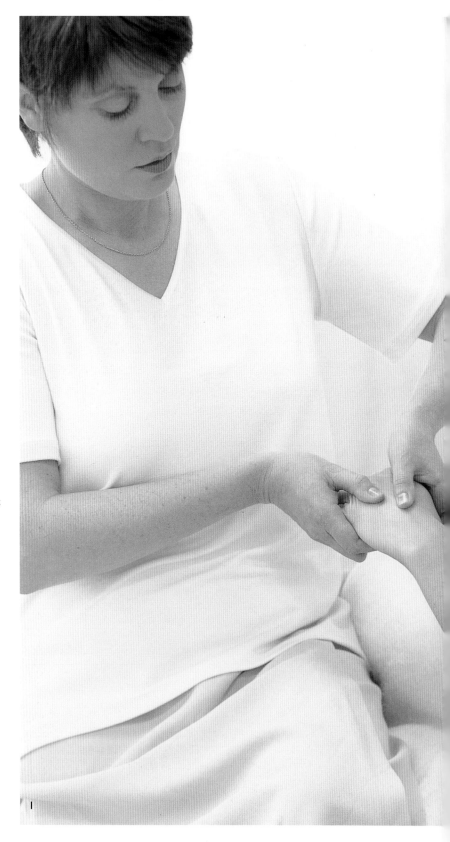

1

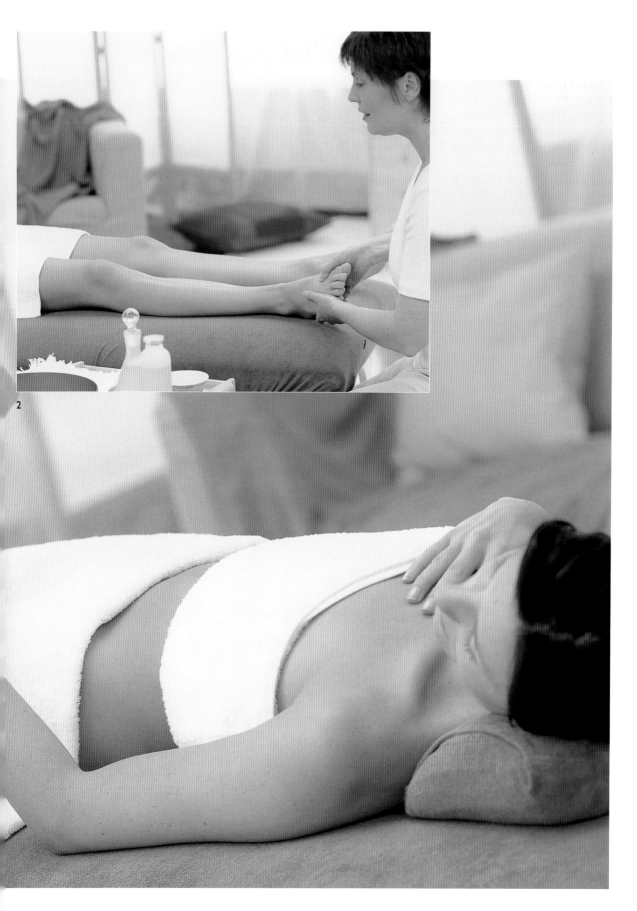

clearing

This is a medium to deep pressure stroke which is used to relax pockets of tension that can build up around joints and muscles close to the spine. The stroke is usually done with the middle and third fingers, applying pressure reasonably firmly. Once again, the idea is to release tension and stimulate the flow of energy. The joints are affected by continued muscular contraction and are often held in a stiff, locked position. This has an obvious effect on circulation and distribution of energy in the body. Always make sure your movements slide rather than press. Be careful to work very gently if your partner suffers from joint pain of any kind.

1 Shoulder blade

Stand facing up your partner's body and place the arm behind the back. Support the shoulder underneath with one hand and place the other at the top of the shoulder blade. Pull your hand slowly towards you, tracing round the shoulder blade as far as you can. Repeat several times.

2 Ankle

Stand at your partner's feet. Lift and support the ankle with your hands. Trace right round the outside of the ankle with your fingers, applying a slight pressure inwards. Imagine you are releasing tension around the joint. Repeat the movement on the inside of the ankle.

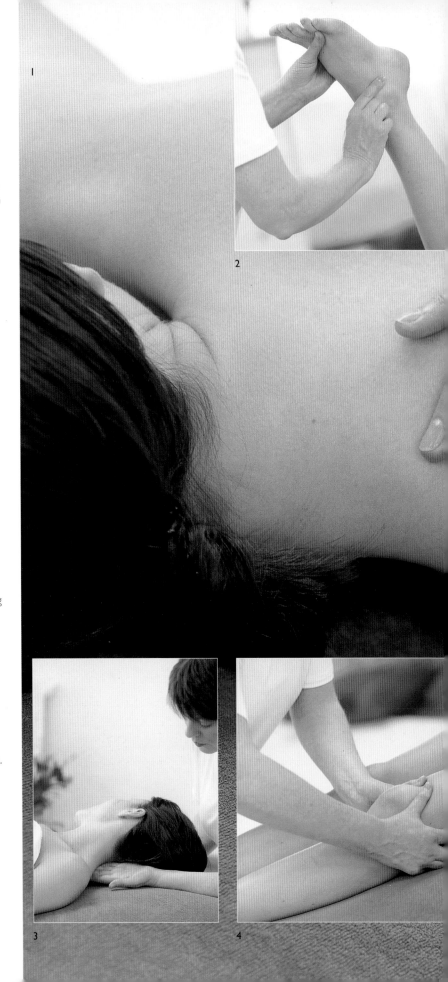

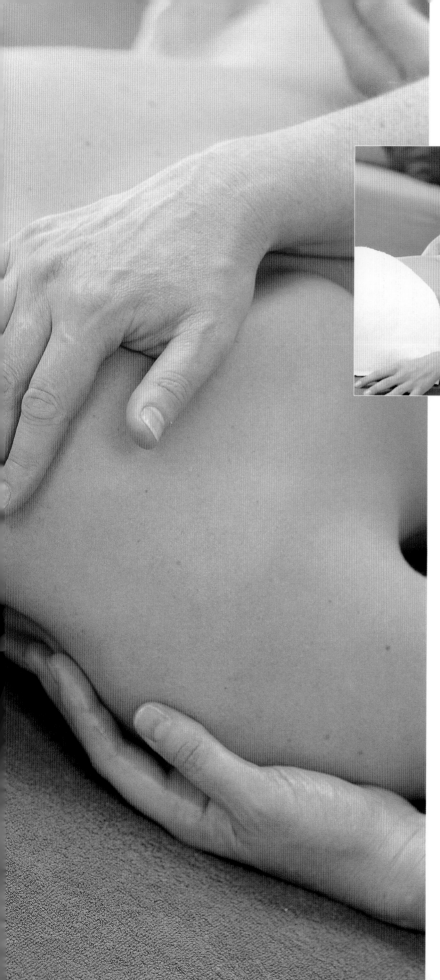

5

3 Neck

Stand at your partner's head. Turn the head to the side and support it in one hand. With the other, reach down underneath the upper back, keeping your fingers close to the spine. Bring your hand back towards you and draw up, along the spine, to the base of the skull. Turn the head the other way and repeat on the opposite side.

4 Knee

Stand at your partner's feet. Place your thumbs just above their knee, with your hands underneath for support. Draw your thumbs around either side of the kneecap until they meet just below it. Now apply a slight pressure inwards. If at any time the knee feels locked, encourage your partner to relax.

5 Ribs

Stand at your partner's head. Reach over the ribcage and place your thumbs between the lower ribs. Slide your thumbs round towards the sides of the body, following the curve of the ribs. Repeat the movement once again further down.

palm sliding

This is a medium pressure stroke using the base of the thumb and palm to slide over the skin. The movement should be smooth, easing tension away from the centre of the body. Palm sliding resembles spreading the thumbs but covers a larger area and allows more pressure from the heel of the hand. Use the stroke where your partner feels particularly tense. Palm sliding is effective when relaxing the back and is especially soothing across the forehead. Imagine you are releasing stress and calming your partner's mind. The sliding movements can also be used working 5 cm/ 2 inches away from the head.

1 Forehead

Stand at your partner's head. Place your palms over the forehead with your thumbs together at the centre. Slide your hands apart towards the hairline, applying pressure with your thumbs as you do so. Repeat the stroke slowly each time, keeping your hands and thoughts relaxed.

2 Upper back

Stand facing up your partner's back. Place your hands between the shoulder blades, beginning the stroke at either side of the spine. Slide your hands outwards to the shoulder blades while applying pressure with the heels of your hands. Repeat the movement slightly further down to release tension in the upper back.

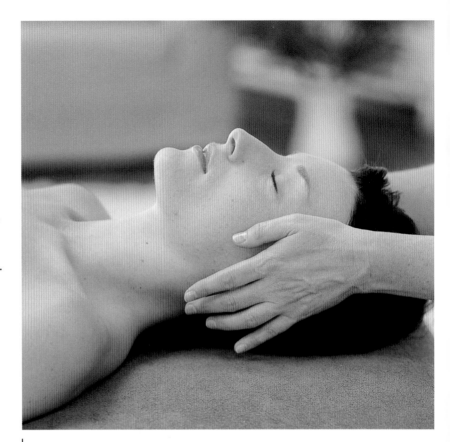

1

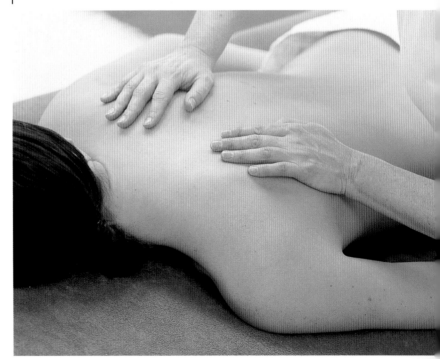

2

draining

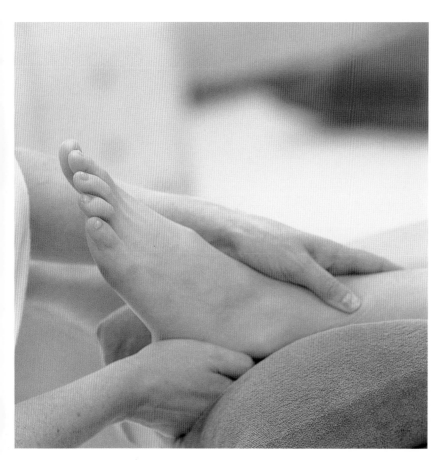

This is a medium pressure stroke which facilitates drainage of the muscles. In the process of relaxing and contracting, the muscles produce waste products which are normally carried away via the blood and lymph. If for some reason this process is restricted, waste products start to build up. Draining along the muscles of the arms and legs is performed towards the body, using the thumbs or whole hand. It can also be used over a smaller area to stimulate local drainage or to help reduce swelling. In the case of swelling, always work away from, and never over, the affected area.

1 Ankle

Facing up your partner's body, support or raise the ankle and place your thumb at least 2 cm/1 inch above any swelling. Gently stroke upwards with your thumb to help reduce the pressure. Work gradually and check that this feels comfortable. If the skin is red to your touch, move further away from the painful area.

thumb and finger circling

This movement is applied to give deep pressure over a particular area by pressing with the thumbs or fingers and making small circles on the spot. As you circle, the pressure continues downwards. Circling can be used, in addition to pressing, over an area where you feel particular tension or a 'knot'. Always check your pressure causes no discomfort or pain. To relax a muscle, begin pressure gently, increasing it when you feel a response. Never force or fight with the muscles. Imagine relaxation radiating out across the body. Circle the area slowly a few times and then move on to avoid resistance or irritation.

1 Sacrum

Stand at your partner's lower back, facing up the body. Reach to the far side of the sacrum (the bony triangle at the base of the spine). Gently press and circle on the spot with your thumb. Repeat across the sacrum, moving out towards the hip. Repeat further down. Imagine you are releasing tension in the lower back and hips.

2 Neck

Stand at your partner's head. Place both hands underneath the neck with your fingers to either side of the spine. Make small circles inwards to the neck and repeat, up towards the skull. If you find it awkward, support the head with one hand and circle one side then the other. Keep your pressure fairly light.

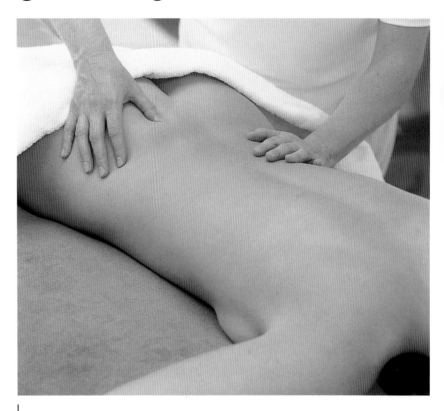

I

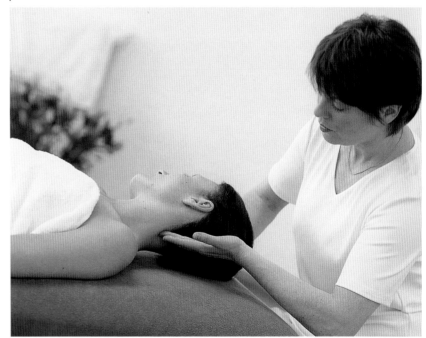

2

thumb press

This movement can be used for deeper pressure to release muscular tension over small areas. It is useful for working on the back, pressing into the muscles on either side of the spine. The pressure penetrates quite deeply, emotionally as well as physically. Press and release smoothly with the balls of the thumbs. Imagine you are releasing tension deep down inside. If you feel resistance, wait until the muscles relax before you continue. Reduce the pressure if you work around the joints and, as always, press very gently over the head and face.

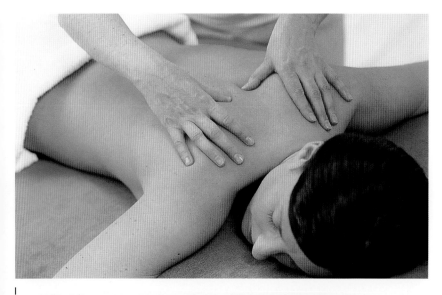

1

1 Back

Relax your arms and place your thumbs at the top of the back, about an inch to either side of the spine. Press down into the muscles once, then release your pressure. Repeat the movement down to the lower back, edging just over an inch lower each time, or pressing approximately once at the side of each vertebra.

2 Forehead

Place your thumbs together above the brows. Press lightly downwards once, then repeat the movement up the centre of the forehead and back towards you. Press to the hairline or to the crown of the head. The slower and more even your pressure, the more effective the movement.

3 Chest

Place both thumbs at the top of the chest, either side of the breastbone. Press slowly and evenly once between the top ribs. Move down between the second pair of ribs and press again. Repeat once, avoiding pressure on the breast tissue. Imagine deep release in the chest.

2

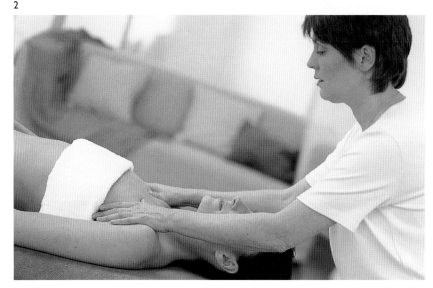

3

opening

This movement helps to prepare the upper back and move the shoulders into a more relaxed and open position before you start work on them. Most of us hold tension in our shoulders. While many people start to relax simply through lying on the table waiting for massage, their bodies, particularly the shoulders, remain in the same contracted position. Part of the function of massage is to restore natural movement. By guiding hunched shoulders into a relaxed position, you are reminding your partner of how their body should actually feel. Perform the movement before massaging the upper back.

1 Shoulder

Stand at your partner's shoulder, facing towards the head. Slip one hand underneath the shoulder and place the other over the shoulder blade. Gently pull towards you, so the body actually moves position. The upper back should then relax. Slide your hands gently away.

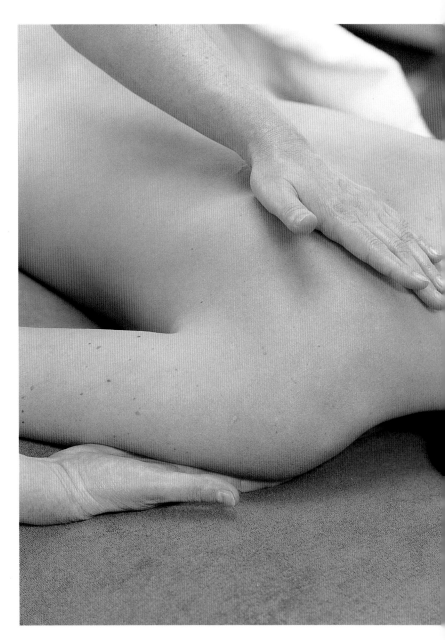

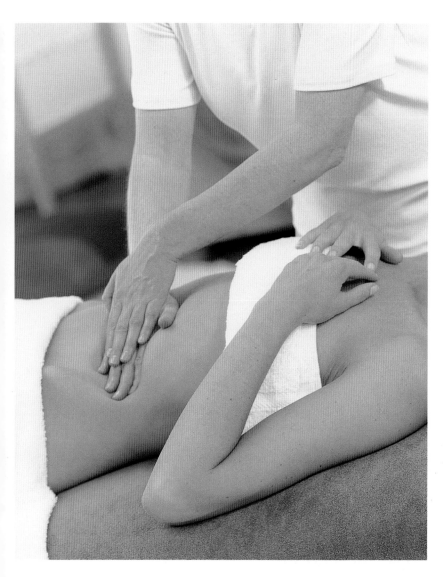

hand press

This is a medium pressure stroke performed just below the ribs. The double-handed action uses the flat of the hand and provides a firm pressure without digging in. It will be more comfortable for your partner if you perform the strokes as they breathe out. Under normal circumstances the pressure will feel good, as it provides an opportunity to reach below the ribs and help stimulate the digestive system. Always make sure you have relaxed the abdominal area first. If your partner has stomach tension or has recently eaten, it is best to avoid this stroke.

1 Abdomen

Stand to the left of your partner, facing up the body. Place one hand over the other, just below the ribs. Press downwards evenly and repeat the stroke twice, moving your hands back towards you. Repeat on the far side of the body, once more moving outwards under the ribs.

diagonal sweep

This is a medium pressure stroke, moving the hands diagonally over the skin to provide a stretch. The stroke is good for stretching the lower back and can be used more gently to stimulate and relax the abdomen. Time your strokes over the abdomen so your hands move as your partner breathes out. Once again, these stretches encourage contracted muscles to relax and give the sense that the body is opening out rather than being held in. Let your hands glide away from each other rather than pressing inwards. Always do the strokes after you have done some initial work to relax the area.

1 Abdomen

Stand facing up your partner's body. Place both hands together over your partner's abdomen. Wait until your partner breathes out and then apply slight pressure with the flat of your hands. Draw the hands diagonally apart to the ribs and opposite hip. Repeat the other way. Stretch outwards to relax the area rather than digging in.

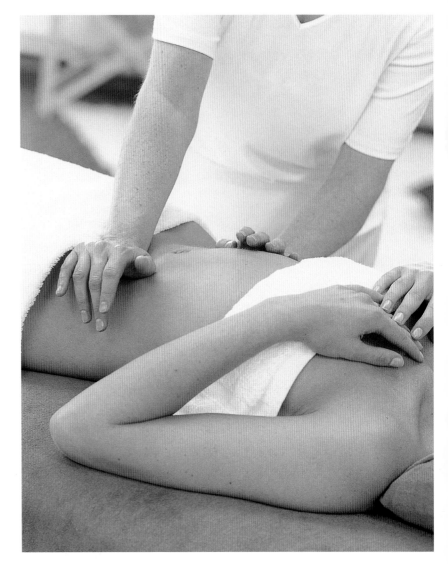

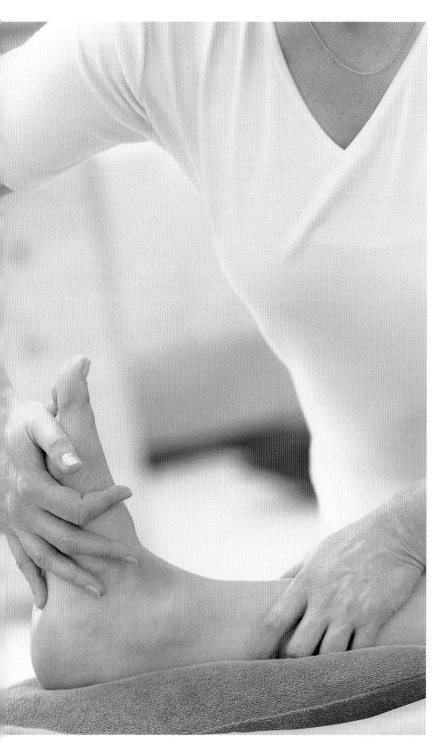

flexing

Flexing is a movement which decreases the angle of a joint, bringing a limb back towards the body or bending the trunk over towards the ground. This particular movement flexes the ankle by pressing back the foot. It helps to make the joint more mobile while at the same time providing a stretch down the hamstrings at the back of the leg. Perform the movement gradually. When flexing the foot the leg lies flat so pressure should be applied slowly in line with the knee. Sharp pain at the back of the leg may be an indication of sciatica or problems in the lower back, in which case you should not continue. Flexing may also be performed on the wrist, with the arm bent and the forearm slightly raised.

1 Foot

Stand facing down the body, towards your partner's feet. Place one or both hands on the sole of the foot and carefully press backwards. Do this gently to make sure there is no discomfort and then repeat, increasing the angle of the foot. Imagine you are releasing tension and encouraging flexibility.

rotating on the spot

This movement can be performed over any area of the body but it is particularly effective over the scalp. The hand is held in a fixed position while the fingers gently rotate on the spot. The pressure remains gentle and rhythmic so the effect is one of relaxation and release. After working over one area, lift your hand away and repeat the movement. Rather than circling movements, which press into the muscles, rotating works lightly over the skin. As you work over the scalp imagine you are releasing mental tension. Use your other hand to lightly support the head.

1 Scalp

Stand at your partner's head. Turn the head slightly and position your hand, with fingers lightly resting, over the scalp. Keeping your hand relaxed, make small circling movements so your fingers rotate over the skin. Lift your hand and repeat the movements until you have covered one side of the head, then complete on the other side with your other hand.

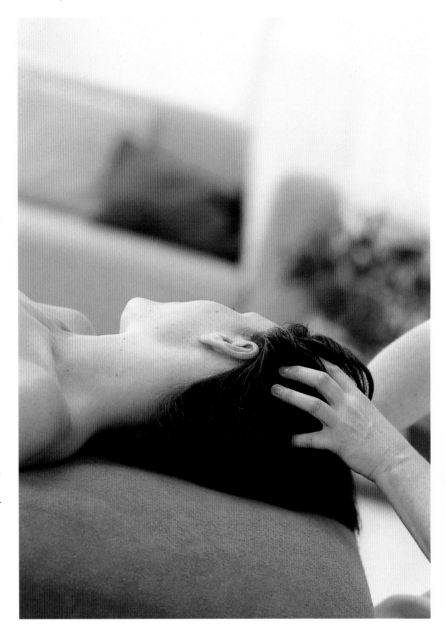

drawing the fingers

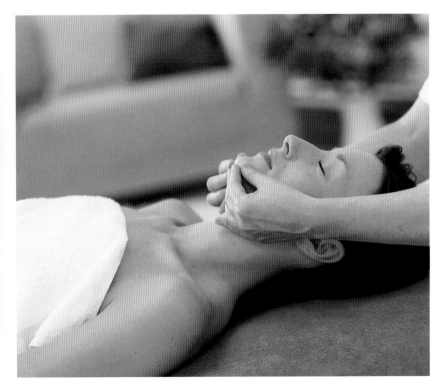

This is a light to medium pressure stroke and is used for delicate movements over the face. Use the balls of the fingers or thumbs to draw over, and just below, the bones. This relaxes the muscles around the brow, cheekbones and chin. If the face is tense it looks heavy, drawn and set. Work outwards and upwards from the centre of the face, taking care not to drag delicate skin.

1 Chin

Place your fingertips together over the chin. Press with the balls of your fingers, along the line of the jaw towards the ears. Press on and underneath the bone. Imagine tension releasing in the face. Repeat slowly, bringing the hands away from the face and up to the ears.

holding

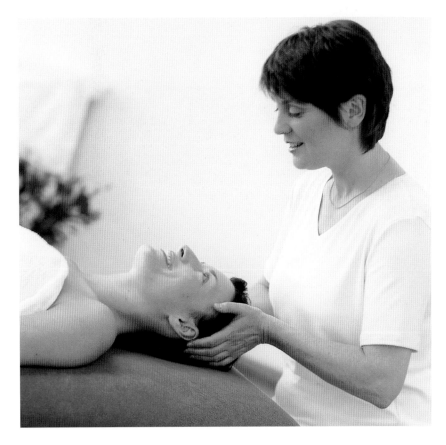

This is a supportive, restful position which can be applied to any area of the body that needs relaxing or where your partner feels emotional or physical pain. Cup your hands gently over the area to provide comfort and allow the body to rest. The warmth of your hands will soothe. Relax your mind and imagine your energy flowing through your hands, even though your body is still. When you feel a change, take your hands gently away.

1 Head

Cup both hands around the sides of the head without applying pressure. Relax your arms and hands and simply rest there. Feel your partner's body relax. Breathe out as you move your hands away.

fanning

This is a light to medium pressure stroke for the back and chest which spreads out from the centre like a fan. The strokes are quick and light with the hands fanning outwards alternately. These strokes not only work physically, they also encourage the body to relax through suggestion. Use your fingertips on the chest and your whole hand over the back.

1 Chest

Place your first two fingers at the top of the chest, to the far side of the breastbone. Fan outwards from the centre of the chest, then repeat the stroke towards you with your other hand. Perform the movements lightly several times, imagining you are opening out the upper chest.

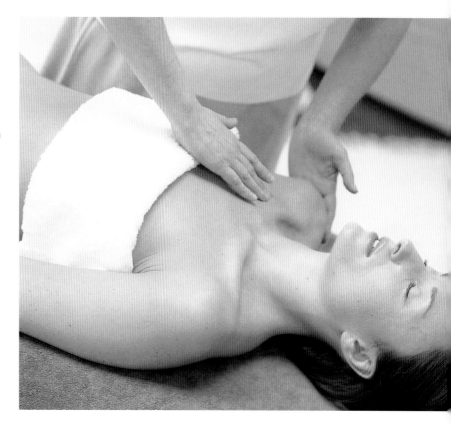

heel press

This stroke uses medium to deep pressure with the heel of the hand. The movement can be performed over the hips, buttocks and the top of the chest. Press into the body and either slightly upwards or away from you. The firm pressure reaches deep into the muscles. Press until you feel a change, check there is no discomfort. Imagine you are helping your partner let go deep inside.

1 Chest

Place the heels of your hands at the top of the chest, just beneath the first rib. Feel for any stiffness. Press down into the chest and slightly away from you. Move your hands outwards and press once again until the muscles relax. Release the pressure evenly.

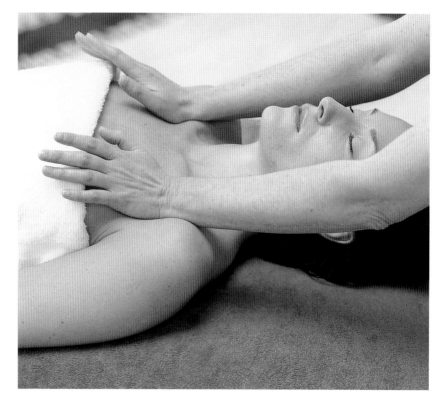

pressing the length of the thumbs

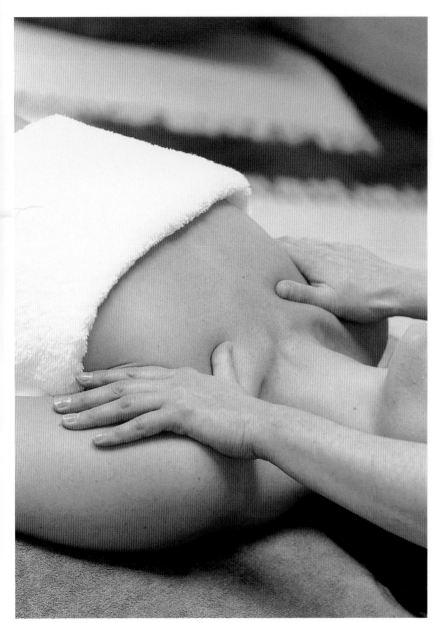

This is a medium pressure stroke and is a variation on thumb pressing. Here, you press with the length of the thumbs, which works particularly well between the ribs. Using the length of the thumb, rather than the ball, reduces the pressure and spreads it over a wider area. This feels more comfortable at the top of the chest and reduces the tendency to dig in.

1 Chest

Place the length of your thumbs just beneath the top rib, to either side of the breastbone. Press downwards with both thumbs, then repeat the movement, moving outwards across the chest. Place your thumbs further down and once again press outwards between the ribs.

massage techniques

lift pull

This movement is performed on the arms and helps to provide a stretch in the shoulders and upper back. The arm is first moved away from the body and then pulled upwards and outwards. This helps to relieve neck and shoulder tension and relax the upper back. Letting someone else move our limbs rarely comes naturally. The response is often to pull back in return. Tell your partner what you are going to do and help them to relax as much as possible. Wait until they do. Make sure you open out your own back as you stretch, as this will be better for you and make the movement more effective. If your partner resists, both of you should relax and try again.

I Arm

Stand square on to your partner. Lift the arm with one hand and crook it over yours. Keeping hold of the wrist, smoothly lift your partner's arm upwards, at the same time pulling it slightly towards you. When the movement is completed comfortably, lower the arm and repeat, increasing the stretch.

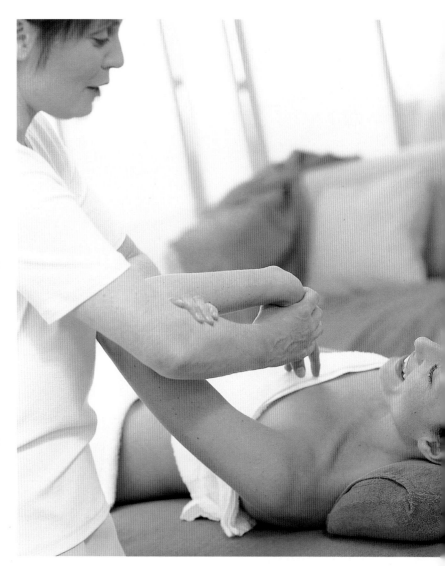

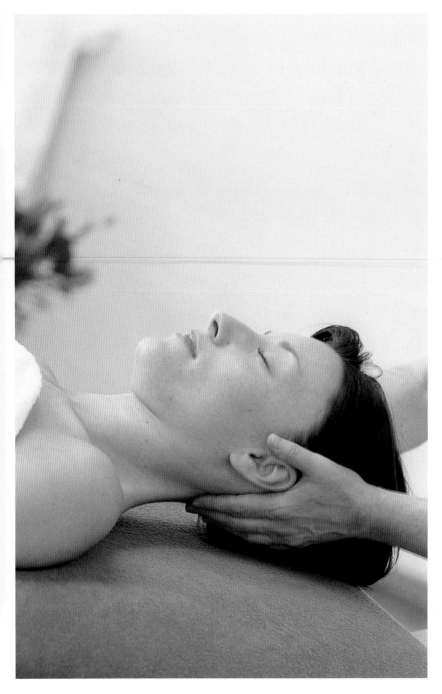

pull

This is a straightforward stretch applied to the legs or neck. Massage is excellent for relaxing contracted muscles but contraction also affects the joints. Stretching helps reduce contraction and increases the flexibility of the back and limbs. After working on the muscles these simple pulls increase circulation and movement and relax the muscles around the joints. Always perform stretches gradually and stop if there is any discomfort. Use your whole body. Make sure you are holding your partner securely and pull evenly towards you, rather than up. Imagine you are releasing energy throughout the body.

1 Neck

Stand or sit at your partner's head and ask them to relax. Cup both hands underneath the neck and pull slowly back towards you. Let your hands slide to the base of the skull. Make sure your arms are relaxed and you are not pulling from the shoulders. Relax, then repeat.

massage techniques

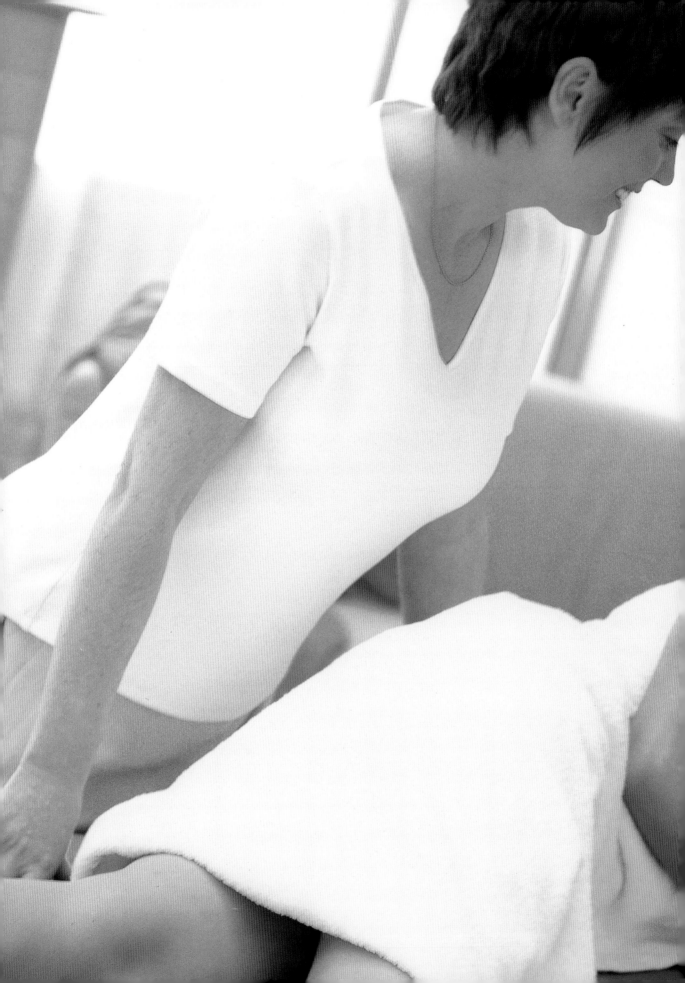

healing massage

This round-the-body massage incorporates the techniques we have discussed, combining massage strokes with healing skills. The attitude and insight that come with healing mean your massage will be different. Healing adds another dimension to massage and speaks directly to the energies of the other person. Listen to your partner, help them to relax and then follow with balancing strokes. As a healing relationship is necessarily dynamic, no two massages will ever be exactly the same. With practice and experience, it is your sensitivity and your partner's needs that will shape the massage.

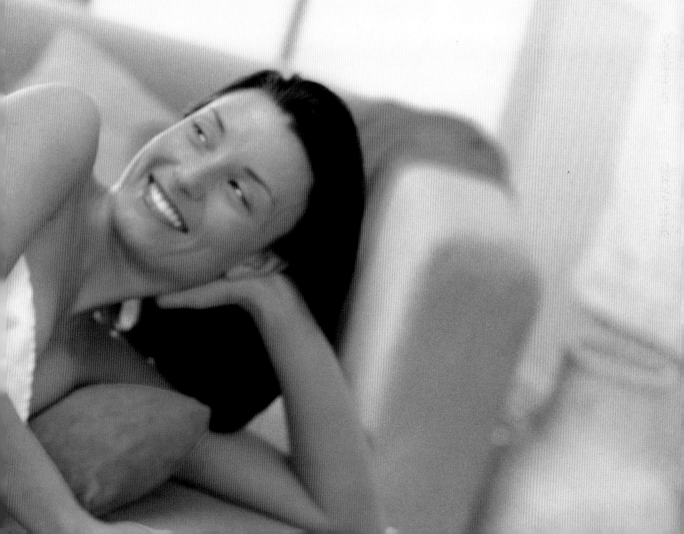

Before beginning, make sure you have all the towels, pillows, oil and warmth you need. Make sure there are no contraindications to massage, (*See page* 7) and note any particular areas of the body that might need special attention. While your partner gets settled, wash your hands.

Step 1

When you are both ready, stand at your partner's head, and make sure you are relaxed and comfortable. Breathe into your abdomen and, as you breathe out, feel the energy move in to your hands. They will probably tingle. Place them gently on your partner's upper back and rest for a moment, noting any sensations or impressions.

Step 2

Move to the lower back, rub a little oil on to your hands and begin gentle effleurage strokes, working up towards the shoulders and returning to the lower back. Apply more pressure on the upward sweep. While you relax the surface of the muscles, make a note of any areas that may need more attention later.

Step 3

Once your partner has begun to relax, you can move to the upper back and shoulders. The massage begins at the top of the back (where most people carry their tension) then works downwards to the feet so your partner will feel centred. Work first on one shoulder, making sure the head is turned away from you. To open out the upper back, place one hand beneath the shoulder with the other on top. Pull gently towards you, encouraging your partner to relax.

Step 4

Now gently knead around the line of the shoulder blade, again coaxing the muscles to soften and relax.

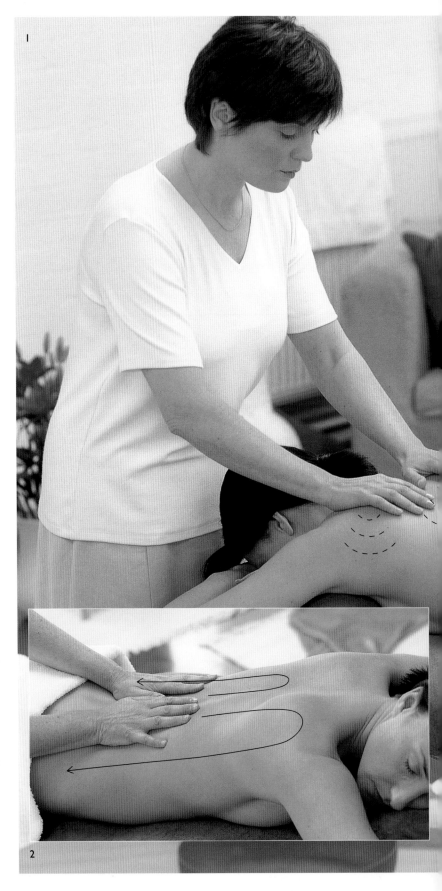

1

2

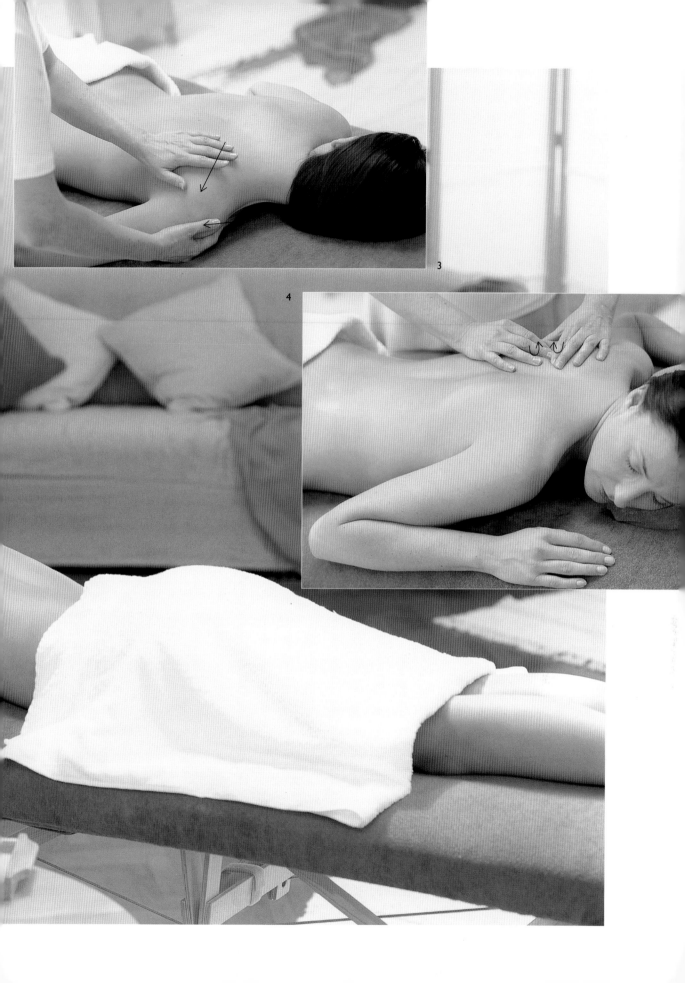

3

4

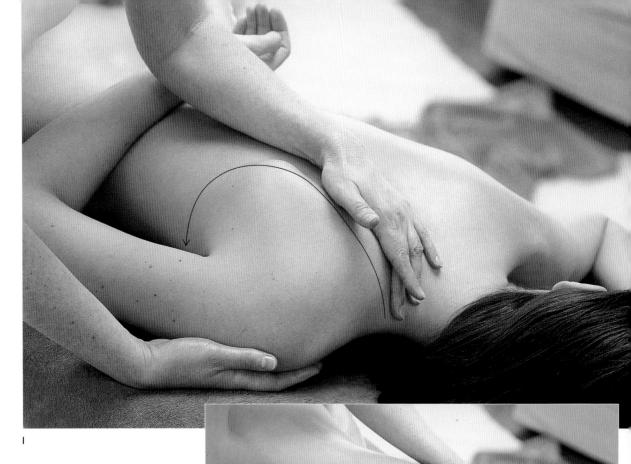

1

The shoulders are a very sensitive area for most people. Typically, it is where we carry physical tension, but this area can also be very emotionally charged. While the massage seems light and gentle, don't underestimate its effect. For some people it can be sheer bliss to let someone else soothe away their tensions; for others it can be quite overwhelming. Always begin your strokes lightly so you can gauge your partner's reaction.

Step 1

To continue the relaxation sequence on the shoulders, place your partner's arm behind their back, and draw round the shoulder blade with your fingers. Begin lightly, then repeat quite firmly, always reducing the pressure towards the arm. Use soothing, sweeping strokes the length of the arm and then turn the head, move to the other side and repeat on the other shoulder.

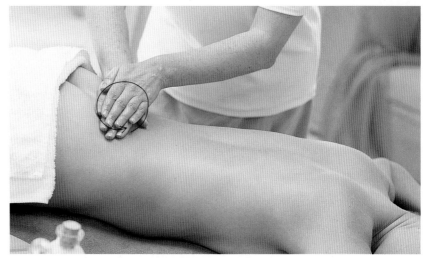

2

3

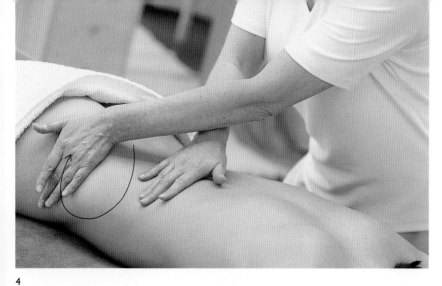

4

Step 2
To finish on the shoulders for the moment, place your hands together between the shoulder blades and slowly slide them apart.

Step 3
Now move to your partner's lower back. Rub some oil between your hands and effleurage over the lower back and hips. Place your hands together over the sacrum and circle slowly in an anticlockwise direction. This soothing, releasing stroke focuses attention on the lower body. Be sure not to use too much pressure.

Step 4
From here, sweep away over the hip and buttock, working away from you to the far side of the spine.

Step 5
Knead any tight muscles around the hips and buttocks.

Step 6
Now circle lightly outwards over the sacrum. Remember, this area can also be emotionally charged.

5

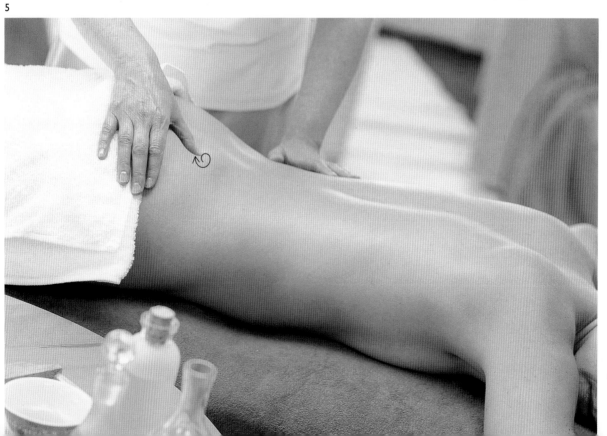

Having worked on the upper and lower back, the next few strokes are aimed at giving a sense of completion and wholeness. As muscles release, so circulation, sensations and energy start to flow. What previously felt like an isolated, stiff shoulder or disconnected, aching lower back begins to feel like part of a whole body that actually belongs together. Bear this in mind as you work on your partner and draw the sense of relaxation downwards through the body.

Step 1

Repeat the sweeping strokes to the far side of the spine but now work upwards from the lower back to the shoulders. Apply pressure as you sweep out over the muscles, at the same time keeping your movements rhythmic. Perform these strokes several times.

Step 2

Gently knead the bands of muscles at the side of the spine. Begin once more at the lower back and work upwards to the neck. Then press your thumb into the muscle band, working downwards from just below the waist. Move to the far side of your partner and repeat the lower back sequence on the other side.

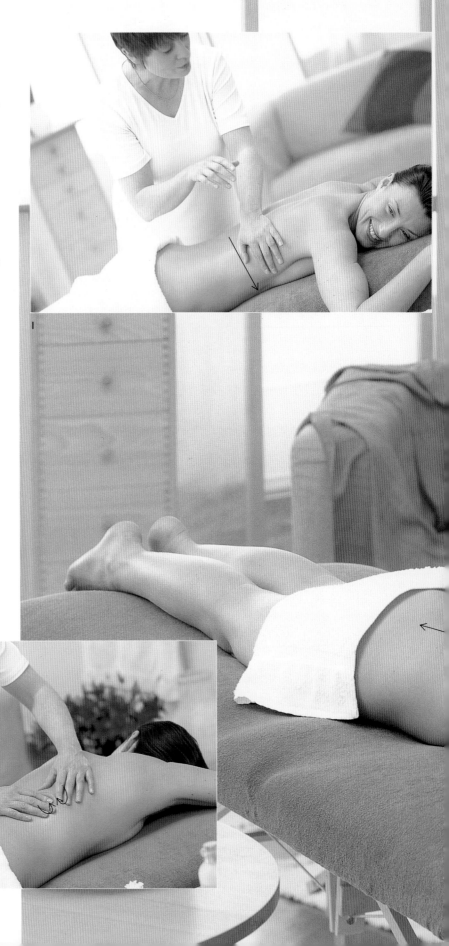

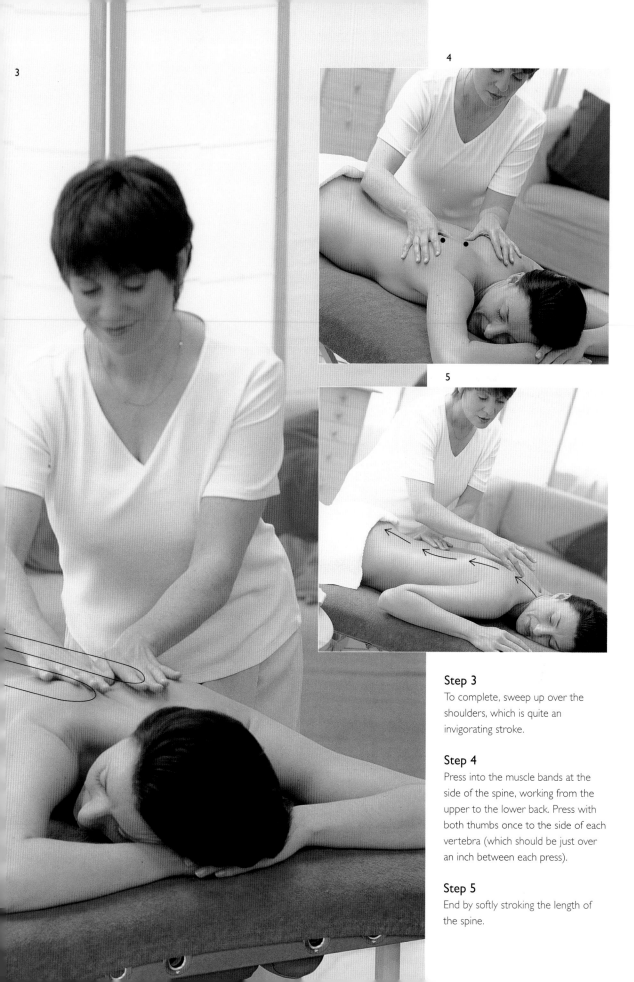

3

4

5

Step 3

To complete, sweep up over the shoulders, which is quite an invigorating stroke.

Step 4

Press into the muscle bands at the side of the spine, working from the upper to the lower back. Press with both thumbs once to the side of each vertebra (which should be just over an inch between each press).

Step 5

End by softly stroking the length of the spine.

If your partner feels receptive and the back is relaxed, you can now try some healing techniques. In truth, there is no real division between the phases of the massage, as we have already seen that massage itself is a healing technique. However, having done some work on physically releasing the body's tension and establishing contact and a relationship between each other, you will find that your partner is more receptive to subtle energy movements, and this in turn is easier for you.

Step 1

Standing firmly balanced and square to your partner, bring your hands over your partner's body, one hand over the upper back and the other over the lower back. Hold your hands roughly 5–15 cm/2–6 inches over the back, noting any particular sensations.

1

2

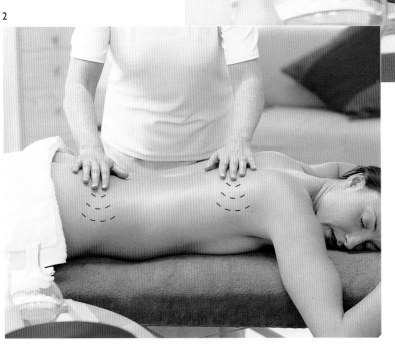

Step 2

Slowly and steadily lower your hands until they rest lightly over the spine. One hand should be just below the shoulder blades, the other over the sacrum. Feel energy flowing through your hands. Rest for a few moments and then make a mental note of any sensations you experience in the lower back, such as warmth, coldness, dullness, tingling or agitation.

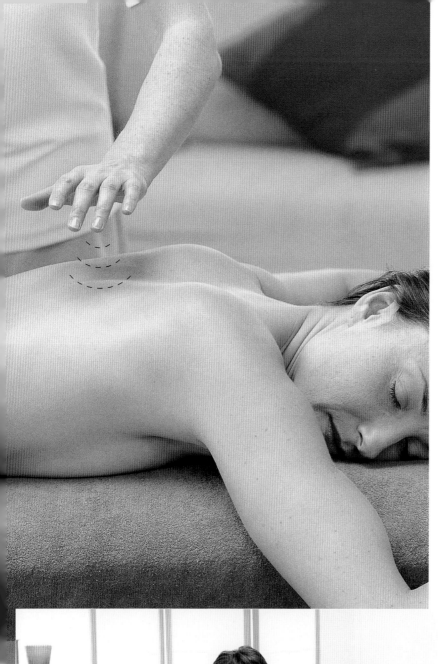

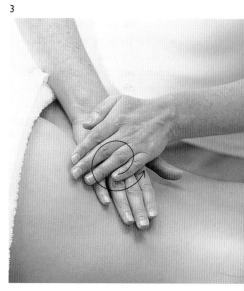

Step 3

To centre your partner, imagine energy gradually moving from your upper hand to the lower back, then circle the sacrum as before.

Step 4

Before starting massage on the legs, place one hand over the sacrum and the other hand over the foot, and imagine energy flowing down the leg. Repeat over the other foot.

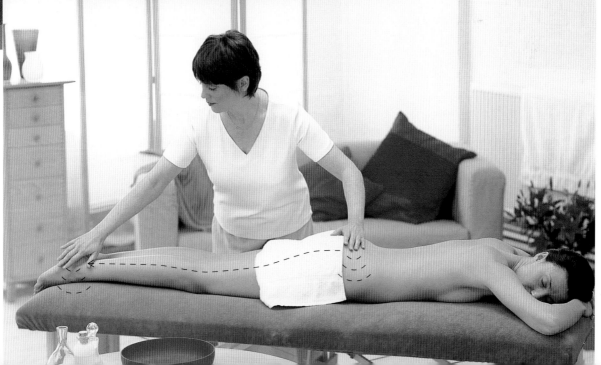

Before starting work on your partner's legs make a note of anything that strikes you. Pay attention to skin tone, shape and whether the feet are warm or cold. You might ask if your partner takes regular exercise to ensure there are no knee or ankle problems. As most of these techniques are working around the joints there is no need to use a lot of oil. However, rub a little on your fingers to give some 'slip', and a small amount over the feet. Although it does not apply to this particular sequence, for future reference only ever brush lightly over varicose veins. Complete all the movements over one leg first, with the idea of directing attention down the body, through the legs and to the feet. It is surprising how few people pay attention to this area of their bodies, and how different an increase in sensation feels.

Step 1

To relax the muscles and joints and release tension in the feet, reach up and rock the leg between your hands, working from the thigh to the ankle. This invigorates and energizes. Find a good position to avoid straining your back and move down the body as your hands complete the movement.

Step 2

Spread your thumbs over the back of the knee. This is deeply soothing and can be repeated several times.

Step 3

Finally, relax the tendon at the back of the ankle by using a plucking movement between the fingers and thumbs. Use your hands alternately and make these movements quick and light.

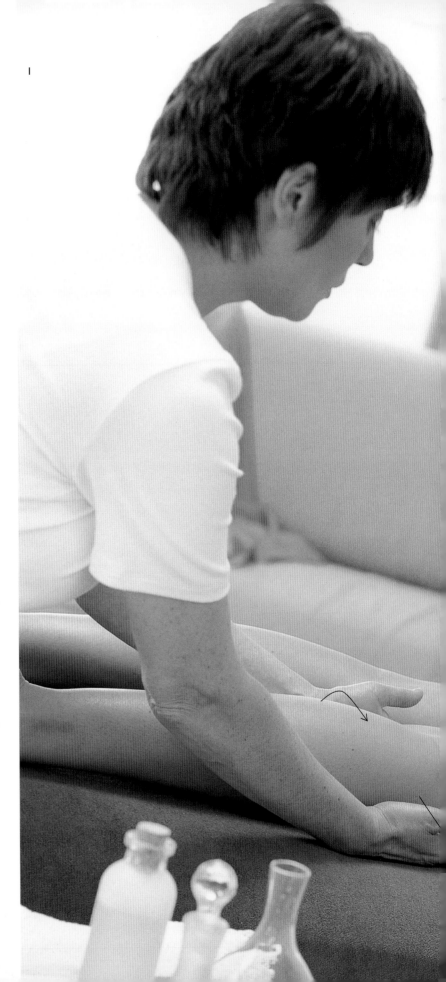

1

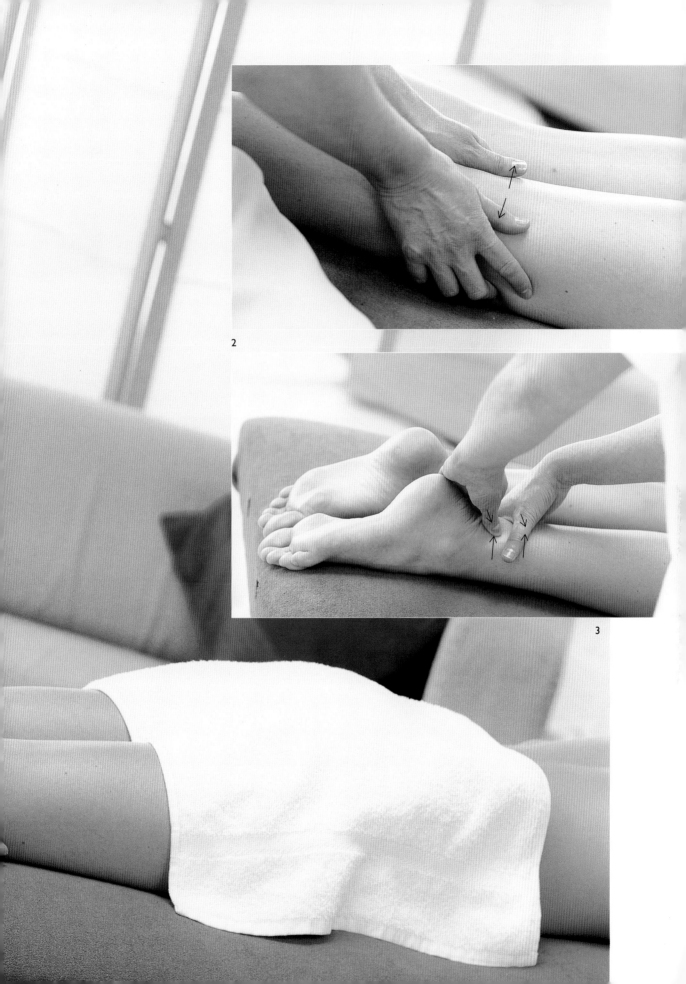

2

3

Massaging the feet not only helps the relaxation process, it also stimulates the body. As the muscles relax and come to life, your partner will become centred and firmly grounded. Although we are pretty good at thinking, curiously, most of us have little awareness of what goes on beneath our feet. Rushing about and raising our stress levels, having an inflexible lower back and stiff knees and ankles can all prevent us from simply having both feet comfortably on the ground.

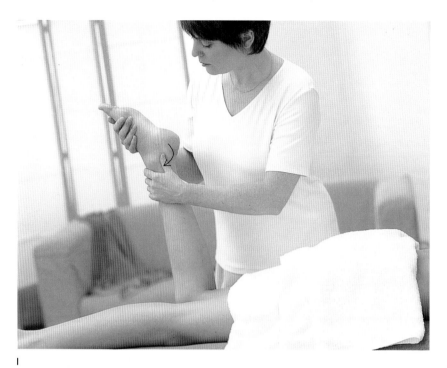

1

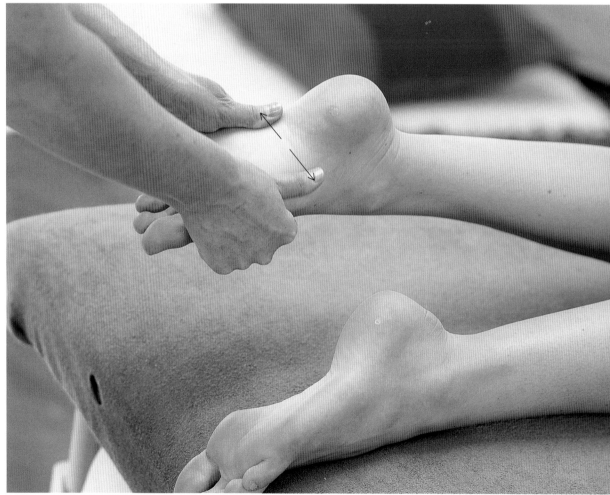

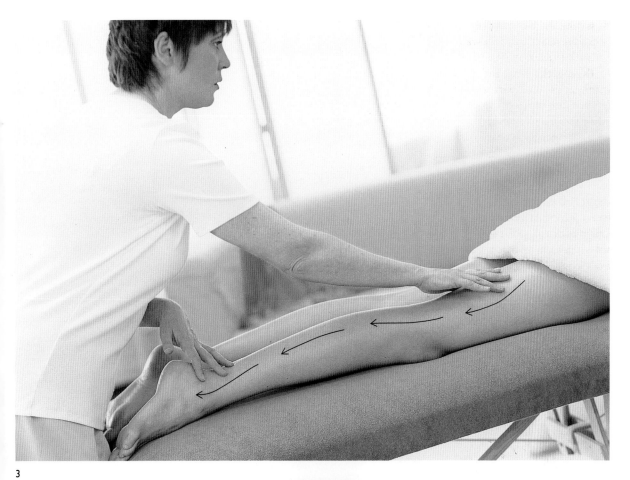

3

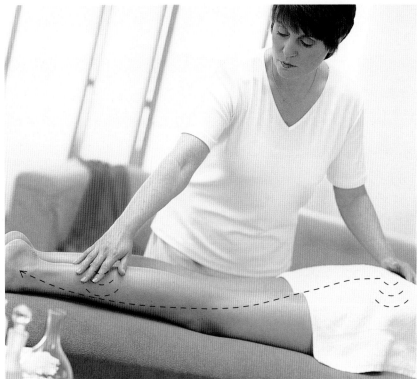

4

Step 1

To continue, support the leg and clear around the ankle joint with fingers and thumb. The pressure can be quite firm, provided there is no tenderness. Remember, you are not simply working on the ankle, you are also increasing circulation and sensation between the legs and feet.

Step 2

Follow with relaxing strokes over the sole of the foot.

Step 3

Stroke lightly over the toes, then repeat on the other leg.

Step 4

Place one hand over the lower back and stroke down the leg to the foot. Repeat on the other side. This movement gives a sense of connection before ending your massage on the back of the body.

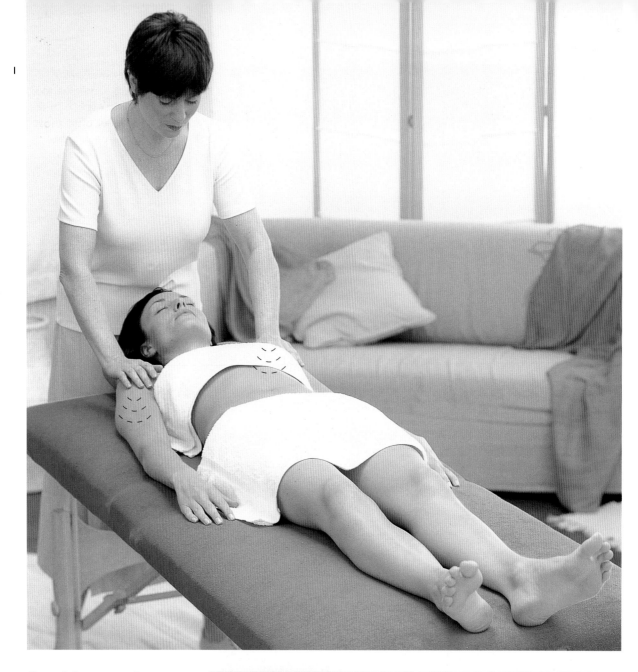

One of the reasons for working on the back of the body first is that it is far less vulnerable than the front. Back massages are fairly common but there is often a feeling of being emotionally exposed when someone is working on the front of your body. This applies to both women and men, so be conscious of this. Your movements will need to be softer on the front of the body. The massage starts at the head and works towards the feet, again so your partner

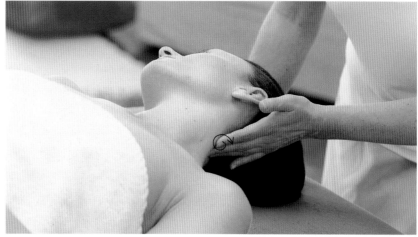

2

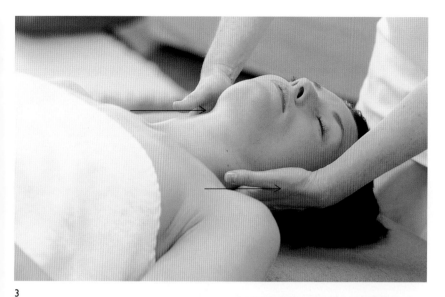

3

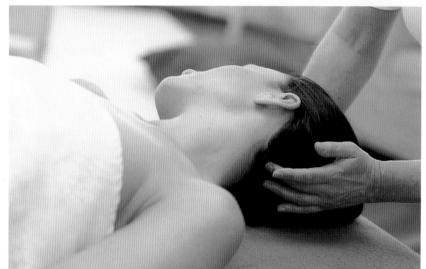

4

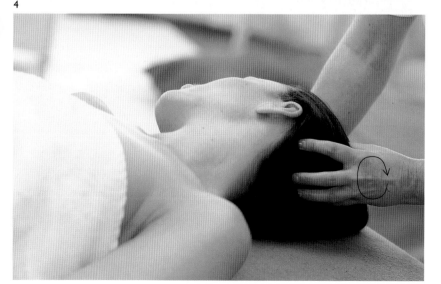

5

ends with a sense of being relaxed, centred and grounded. Relaxing the neck is one of the most valuable, but often most difficult, things you can do. It is common for the neck to be stiff and this is often accompanied by upper back tension and headaches. For some people, giving the weight of their head to another person is almost impossible. Be patient and never struggle with your partner. Wait until they are thoroughly relaxed and ready to receive.

Step 1

Begin by centring yourself. Check that your shoulders have not become tense and that your hands are soft and relaxed. If necessary, take a few moments to shake out your arms. Breathe into your abdomen and then breathe out, placing your hands on your partner's shoulders. Feel the flow of energy through your hands.

Step 2

The first movement involves small circles along the muscles to the side of the spine, working from the base of the neck to the skull. This can be performed with the neck straight or turned to one side.

Step 3

Follow this by a relaxing stretch.

Step 4

Turn the head and press just below the base of the skull, in a line out towards the ears.

Step 5

Rotate your fingers over the scalp. Repeat on the other side.

Face massage is deeply releasing and relaxing. Faces – and backs – tell a good deal about a person. These muscles are generally working every minute of the day and are what we use, literally, to face the world. The eyes take and give out energy, while the skin reflects our various emotional states and experiences of environmental stress. As the skin is so delicate, make sure you work from a steady position so that you do not lean on your partner or drag on the skin. A stool or cushion often helps. If your partner's skin looks particularly tight or dry, rub a little oil between your hands, and apply a small amount to the face.

Step 1

To relax the forehead and soothe mental stress, begin by gently pressing the balls of both thumbs up the centre of your partner's forehead. Work up to the hairline, repeating several times.

Step 2

Smooth over the forehead, this time with the length of the thumbs.

Step 3

Follow with slightly deeper pressure, using the palms and heels of the hands. The hands should slide over the area, without pulling.

Step 4

Trace over the eyebrows towards the temples, pressing with the balls of your fingers. All these movements should be quite delicate, with the idea of drawing tension away from the centre of the face. As you will notice, there are only very small, but important, differences in the positions of your hands.

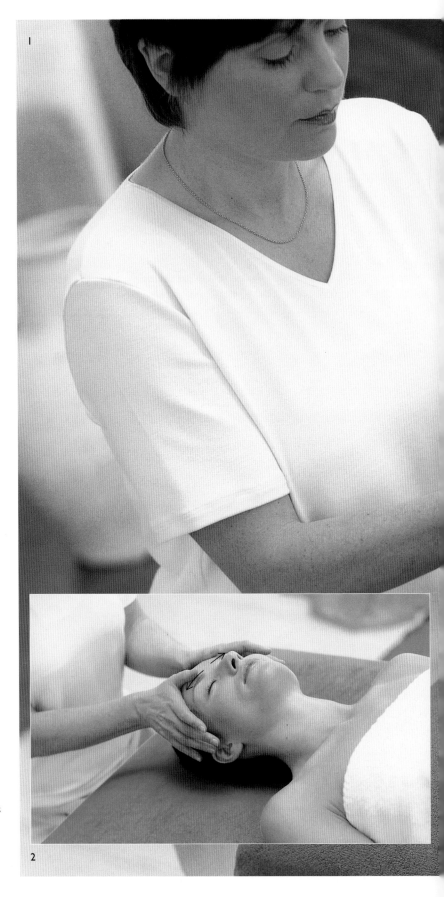

1

2

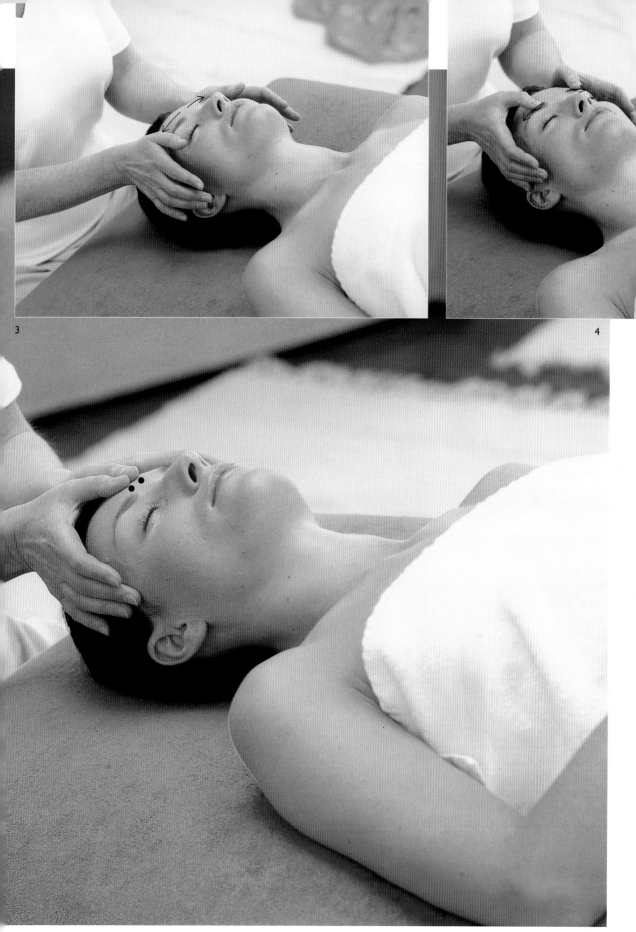

Faces reflect stress. A grimly set face has a story to tell and the effects can often be seen, and certainly felt, around the cheeks and jaw. To work on the face you must strike a balance between using light, uplifting movements, making sure you do not drag the skin, and being firm enough to be effective where needed. Always end the movements in an upwards direction, as this lightens the face and encourages smiles. If the teeth are clenched you can point this out, and suggest that your partner drops their jaw a little. Take a moment to relax your shoulders, shake out your hands if necessary, and resist the temptation to be drawn in towards the massage surface. Make sure you have enough oil on your hands and remember to keep them relaxed.

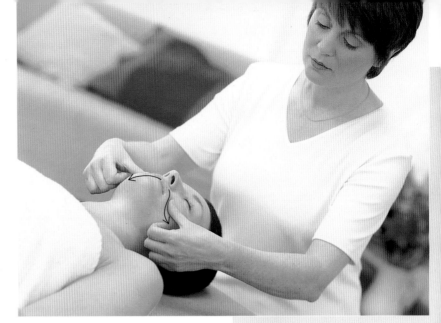

I

Step 1
Draw the balls of your thumbs over the cheeks and under the cheekbones several times.

Step 2
Press gently but firmly with your fingertips, in a line from under the cheekbones towards the ears.

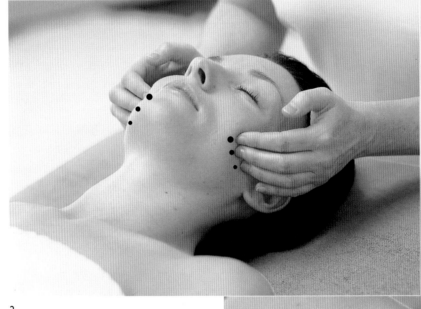

2

Step 3
You can then help release the muscles around the jaw by making loose circles towards you with your fingertips. If you are unsure where to perform the movements, ask your partner to open and close their jaw to see how the muscles move.

Step 4
Help to relax the jaw further by drawing outwards from the centre of the chin up towards the ears, making a light squeezing movement. End by pressing, gently but firmly, once above the upper lip, and once in the hollow just above the chin.

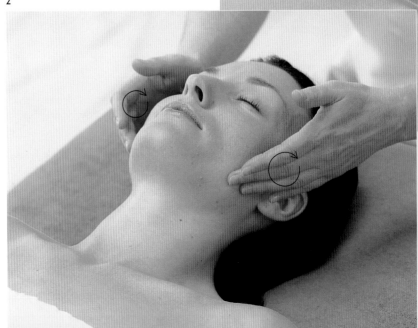

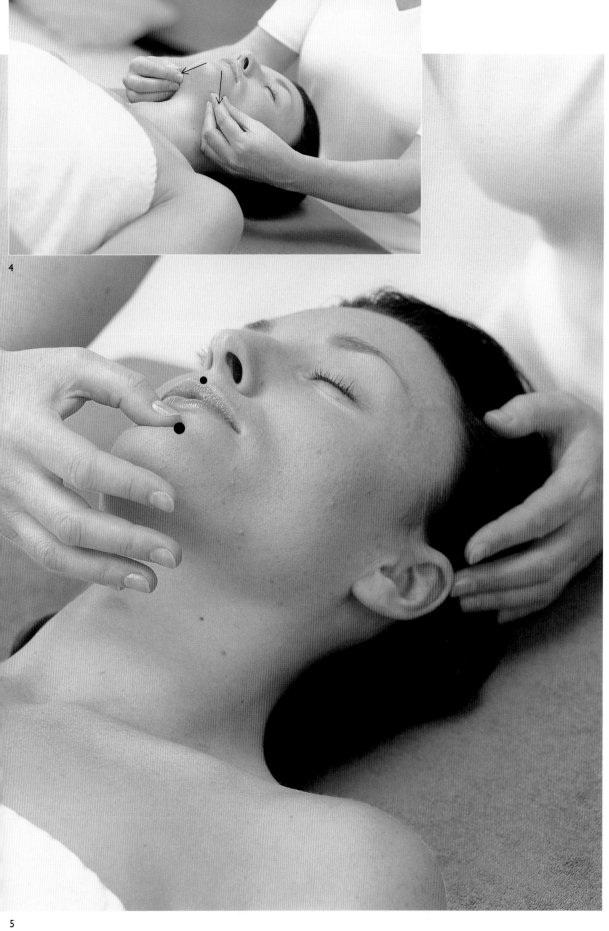

4

5

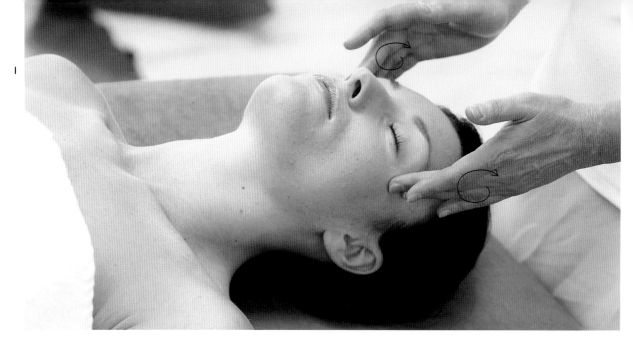

1

This sequence completes the massage over the face and head. In general, very little healing work is done over the head. The head and face are particularly sensitive and there is often too much activity – usually of the wrong kind! These gentle and soothing techniques should not prompt you to interact with your partner, other than as a supportive, calming presence. Even the most subtle movement can be sensed keenly so it is very important to work with sensitivity. Calm your thoughts, relax your arms and shoulders and ensure your movements are not too close or intrusive. Abrupt movements or hands held too close to the face can be unpleasant, but if done gently, the techniques feel soothing, relaxing and restorative.

Step 1
Bring your hands to your partner's temples and make gentle, slow circles towards you.

Step 2
Stroke over the top of the head.

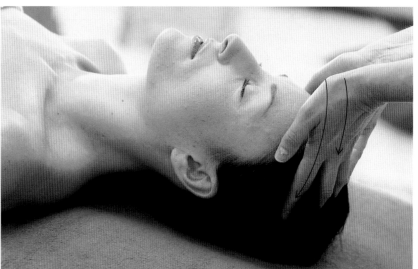

2

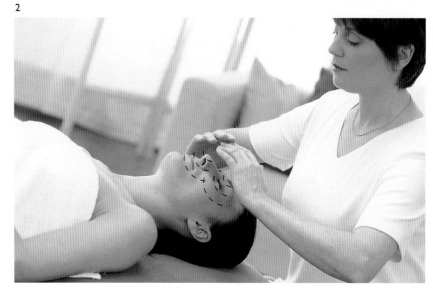

3

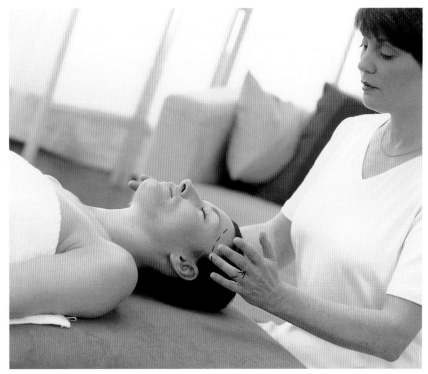

Step 3

Carefully bring your hands up over your partner's eyes and hold them about 12–15 cm/5–6 inches away in that position. This helps rest the eyes. Remember that heat is generated by your hands, so make sure this is a comfortable distance for your partner. Simply rest and breathe.

Step 4

After a few moments, slide your hands, still without touching your partner, to the back of the head.

Step 5

Gently cup your hands around your partner's head and rest for a few moments, experiencing peacefulness. When you are ready, move your hands away again softly.

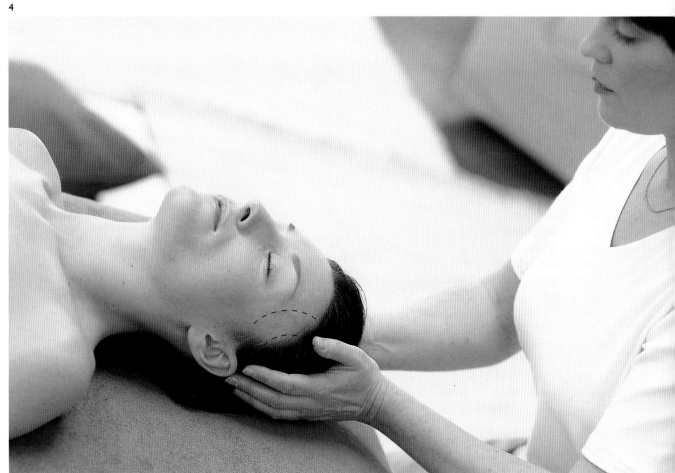

Working over the chest is very important and can have a profound effect. A lot of emotions can be held here and this may go along with shallow breathing and stiffness around the shoulders. Again, the area is extremely sensitive so little direct healing work is done over the chest. The most important thing is relaxation. Your partner's chest needs to be relaxed for there to be a proper connection to the abdomen and arms. Sometimes it can feel a little awkward for your partner. If you are massaging a woman, work down the centre of the chest and keep well clear of the breasts. If your partner prefers to use a small towel, there is no problem working around it. The main thing is for you both to feel comfortable. Remember, always avoid working over the delicate and tender breast tissue.

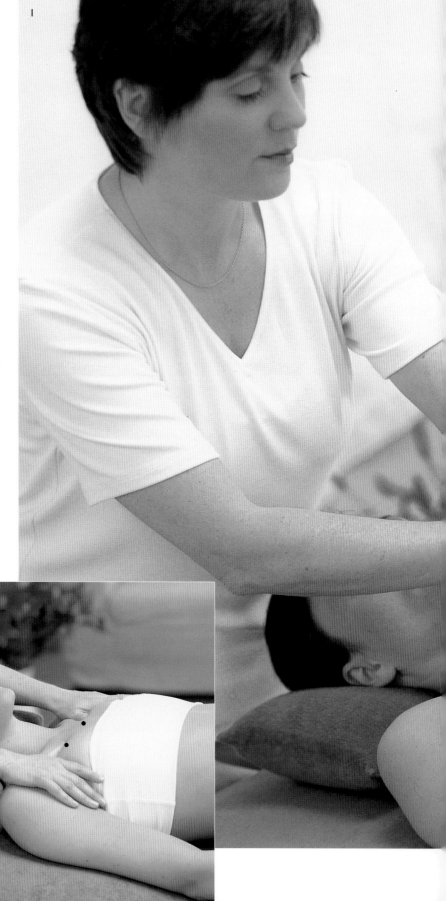

1

2

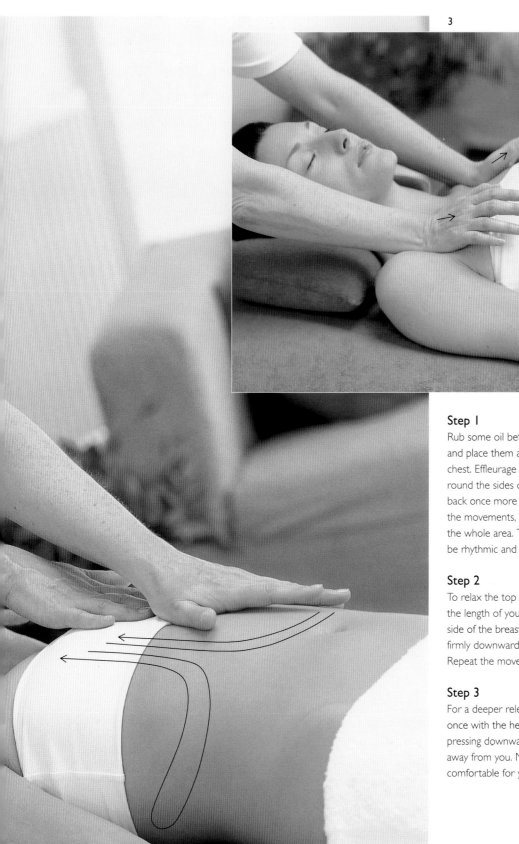

Step 1

Rub some oil between your hands and place them at the top of the chest. Effleurage down the centre, round the sides of the ribcage and back once more to the top. Perform the movements, soothing and relaxing the whole area. The strokes should be rhythmic and sweeping.

Step 2

To relax the top of the chest, place the length of your thumbs at either side of the breastbone and press firmly downwards, then release. Repeat the movements outwards.

Step 3

For a deeper release, press firmly once with the heels of your hands, pressing downwards and just slightly away from you. Make sure this feels comfortable for your partner.

85 healing massage

The following few movements help to relax the muscles between the ribs so that the ribcage can move more easily. Observe the way your partner's body moves as they breathe. When lying flat there should be little movement in the chest and a relaxed feeling in the diaphragm and lower abdomen. Coaxing your partner's shoulders to let go will help relax the chest and encourage natural breathing patterns. My personal feeling is that deep, relaxed breathing happens gradually and naturally, when mind and body are at ease. Focusing on the breath or trying to alter breathing patterns can sometimes be disturbing or may create further tension. Draw your partner's attention to it if you feel the chest area is very tight, and perhaps suggest some relaxation exercises later. You, too, should relax your shoulders and make sure you are also breathing naturally. When you are working so closely with someone it is very easy to pick up each other's habits.

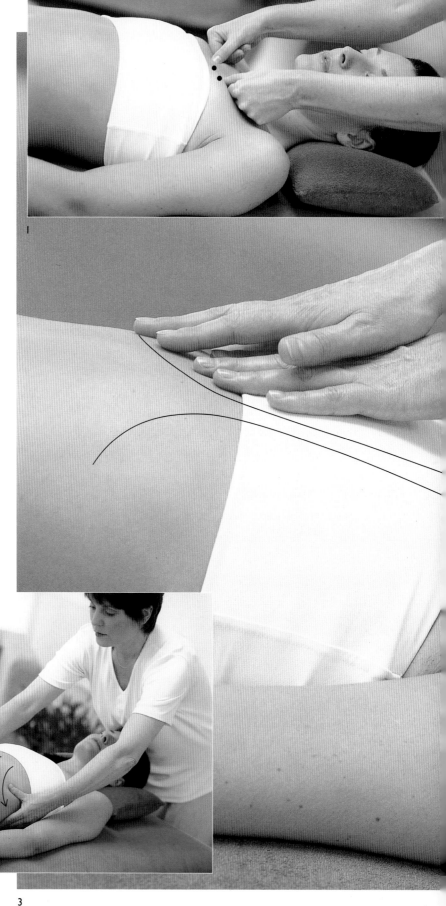

1

2

3

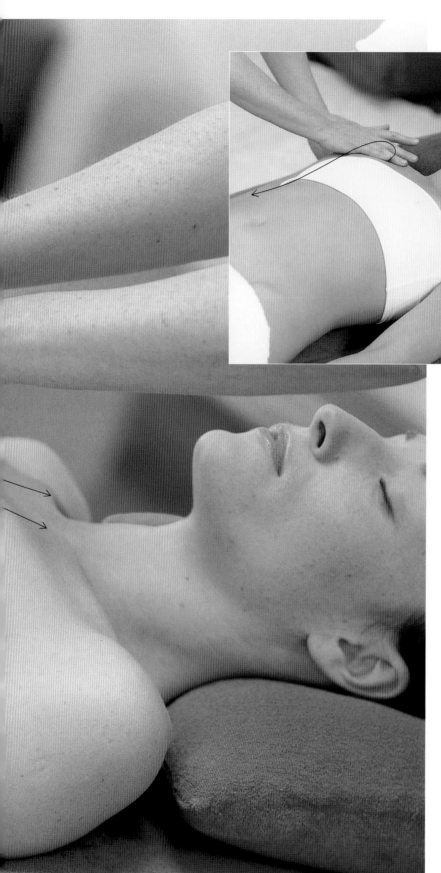

Step 1

Standing at your partner's head, quietly reach over and place your thumbs at the top of the ribcage, on either side of the breastbone. Press between the first two ribs, release and repeat the movements twice, working down the chest.

Step 2

Reach over the ribcage and place your thumbs between the lower ribs. Sweep round to the sides of the body. This movement can be repeated several times over the lower ribcage.

Step 3

Sweep back over the chest.

Step 4

Finally, stroke the length of the arms. These final sweeping and stroking movements help to relax the upper body and make a connection with the arms.

Massaging the arms completes the work on the upper body. Circulation, movement and energy increases when the chest and shoulders are relaxed. Ideally, the arms swing and express themselves without inhibition and feel like an extension of the upper back. Once again, we are going to concentrate on the release around the joints, drawing the attention through the arms to the fingers. You will need to be in a comfortable position. You can support the arms on the elbow while you work, or in your hands. Note any differences between the right and left arm – it is a little like fitting together a fascinating jigsaw puzzle.

Step 1

Rock the length of your partner's arm to release any stiffness. If it is particularly heavy, cupping your hands right underneath to lift the arm will help you. Giving another person the weight of our limbs is always strange the first time, so be patient while your partner relaxes and gets used to the idea.

2

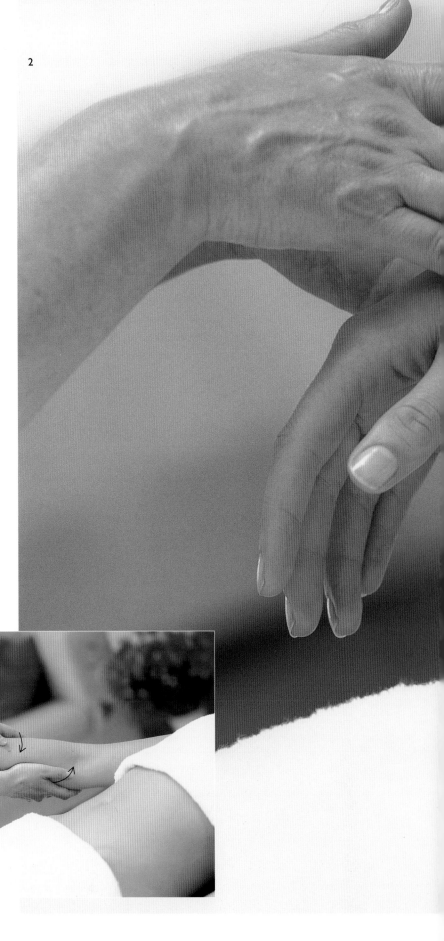

healing massage

1

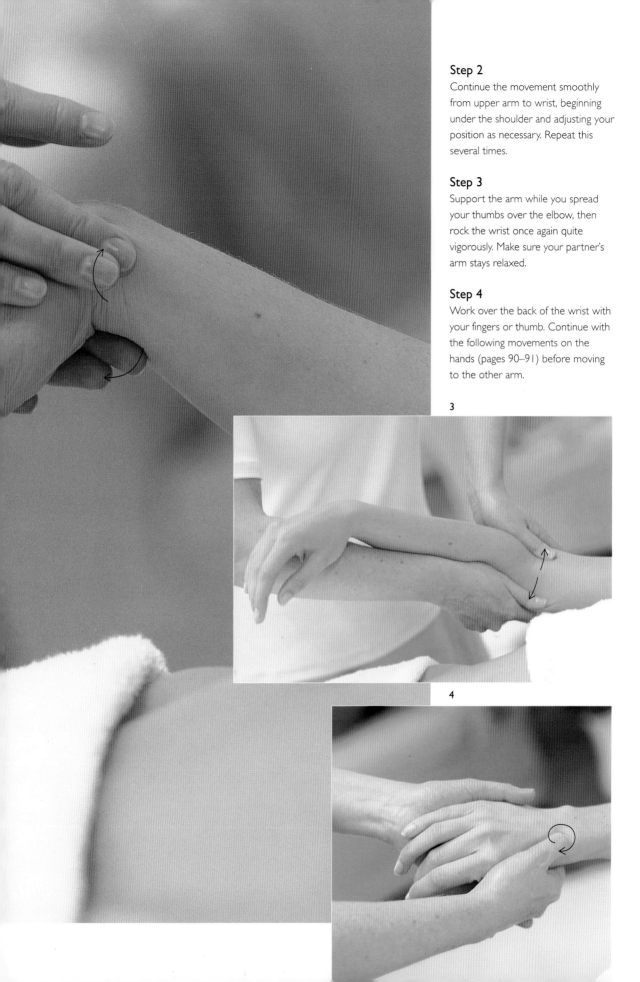

Step 2
Continue the movement smoothly from upper arm to wrist, beginning under the shoulder and adjusting your position as necessary. Repeat this several times.

Step 3
Support the arm while you spread your thumbs over the elbow, then rock the wrist once again quite vigorously. Make sure your partner's arm stays relaxed.

Step 4
Work over the back of the wrist with your fingers or thumb. Continue with the following movements on the hands (pages 90–91) before moving to the other arm.

3

4

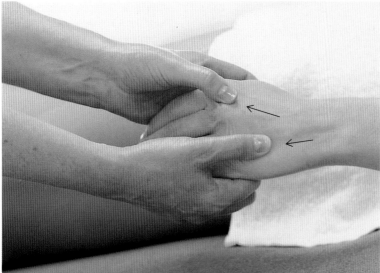

1

Working on the hands soothes and releases. As we use them so much, a quick massage over the hands alone is a wonderful energy restorer. As mentioned before, sensitive energy centres are located here. If you give massage, your hands are your tools, so learn to take care of them. As someone who is using their hands sensitively, you should also develop an interest in those you work on. Rub a little oil over your fingers if necessary, and some over your partner's hand if the skin is dry.

Step 1

Make sure your partner's arm is supported and hold their hand in your own. Begin by drawing down between the tendons, moving outwards across the hand from the thumb. This should give the feeling of release and is a slow, languid stroke you can perform several times.

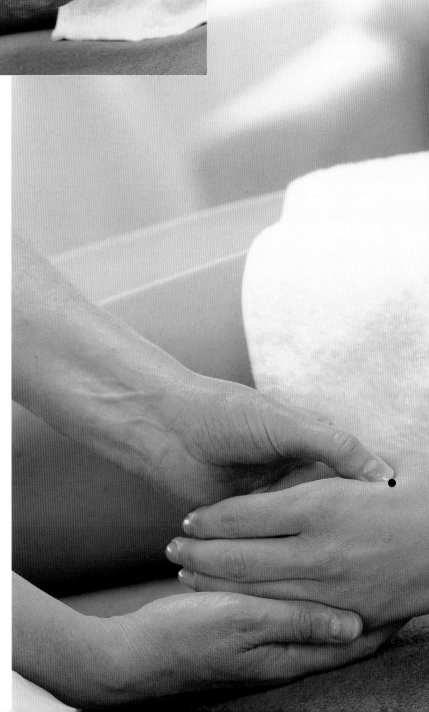

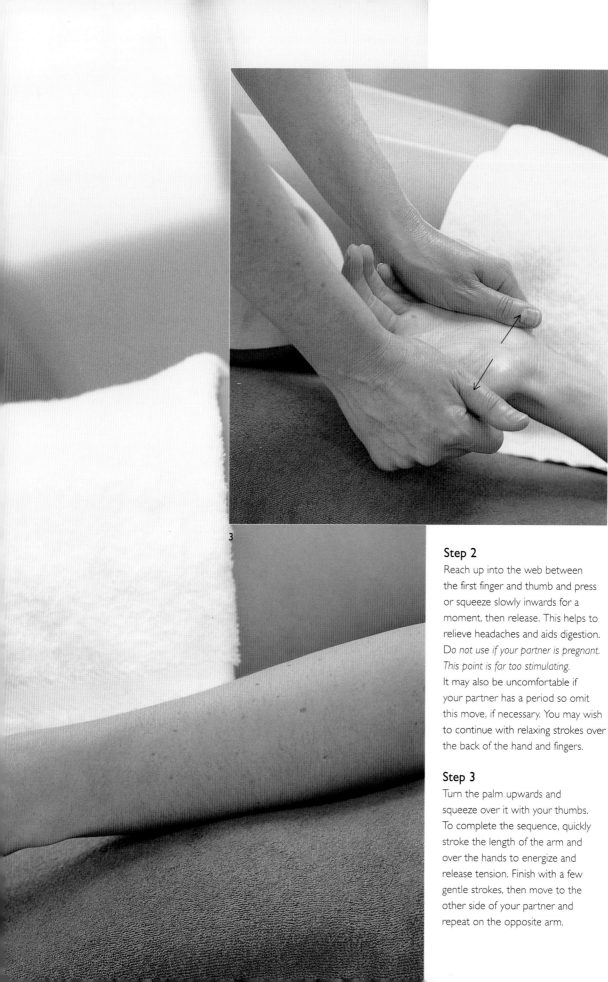

Step 2

Reach up into the web between the first finger and thumb and press or squeeze slowly inwards for a moment, then release. This helps to relieve headaches and aids digestion. *Do not use if your partner is pregnant. This point is far too stimulating.* It may also be uncomfortable if your partner has a period so omit this move, if necessary. You may wish to continue with relaxing strokes over the back of the hand and fingers.

Step 3

Turn the palm upwards and squeeze over it with your thumbs. To complete the sequence, quickly stroke the length of the arm and over the hands to energize and release tension. Finish with a few gentle strokes, then move to the other side of your partner and repeat on the opposite arm.

The abdomen is an extremely
important area of the body,
which is also very sensitive. In-
depth diagnoses can be carried
out from this area. When one
refers to being centred, the
area just below the navel is
the physical location we mean.
The area should feel relaxed
and 'full' and should move as
the body breathes. Once again,
work lightly over the abdomen
to gauge your partner's
reaction, massaging with the
flats of the hands to avoid
uncomfortable digging in.
*Do not massage over the
abdomen during the first four
months of pregnancy – just rest
your hands. After this, perform
the effleurage and gentle circling
movements only.*

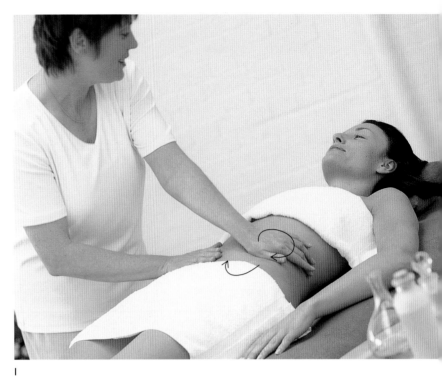

I

healing massage

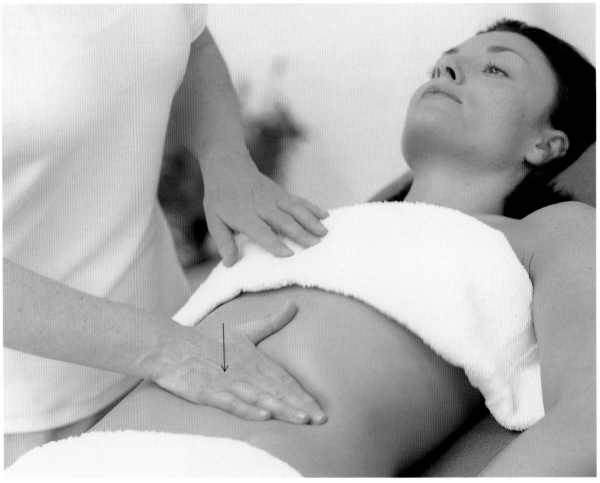

2

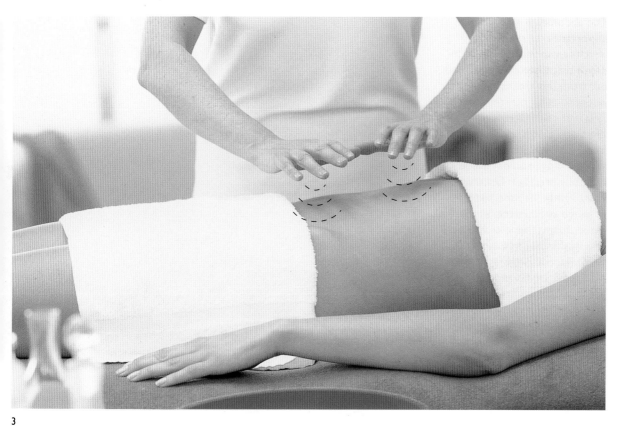

3

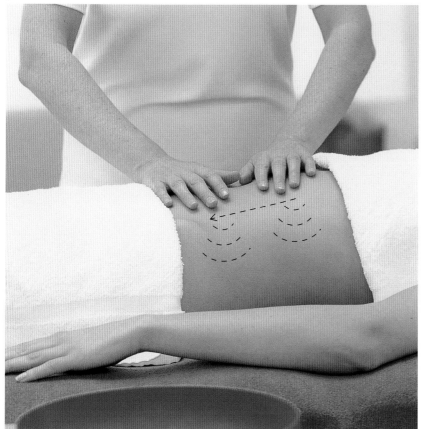

4

Step 1

Rub a little oil on your hands and gently effleurage over the abdomen. With palms flat, make slow circles in a clockwise direction. Always keep one hand in contact with the body. Note any feelings of warmth, cold, tension or bloating and how the abdomen moves as your partner breathes.

Step 2

Put one, or both, hands under the rib-cage. Ask your partner to exhale; press gently but firmly downwards, avoiding the solar plexus. Repeat this further towards you. Reach over and repeat twice on the other side.

Step 3

Centre yourself, calm your mind and hold your hands over the abdomen.

Step 4

Gently lower the hands, resting one below the solar plexus and the other just below the navel. Imagine your lower hand becoming full and then lift your upper hand away.

For the closing sequences of the massage we end by working over the legs and finish at the feet. It is in a sense artificial, although convenient, to look at the different parts of the body separately. At this stage what is important is getting a sense of the whole, and the way each area of the body relates to the rest. The pelvic area, the strength and position of the lower back and the muscles around the buttocks and hips directly affect the legs. If these muscles are relaxed, circulation and flexibility increase. As a general rule, most people need to regain their sense of being comfortable with the ground and able to relax downwards through the body.

Step 1

Begin by encouraging your partner to feel the connection between the abdomen and feet, working over both legs before continuing the sequence. Make sure you are centred and can reach comfortably. Once again, make a note of any particular features about your partner that may strike you at this point.

Step 2

To relax the muscles, shake and rock the leg as before, beginning as high towards the hip as you can. Repeat several times.

Step 3

Draw round the kneecap with your thumbs. Begin gently to make sure there is no tenderness and then repeat more firmly, pressing in very slightly towards the knee.

Step 4

Lightly stroke down the leg and then slowly draw both thumbs around the ankle joint.

healing massage

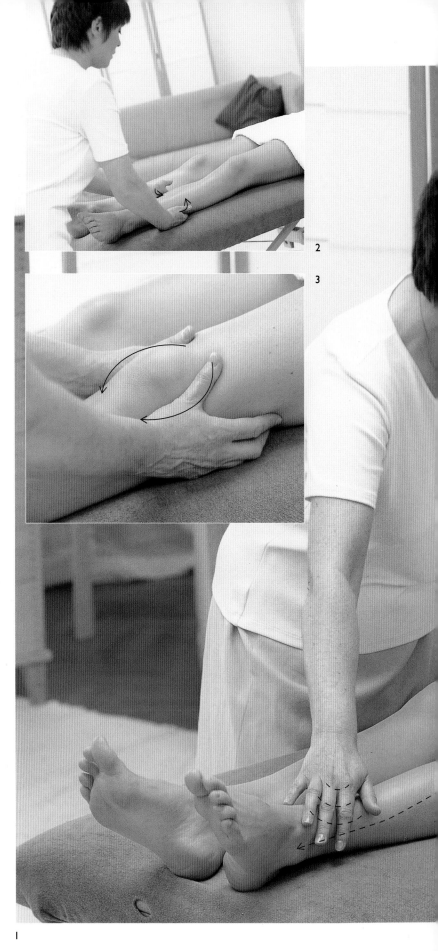

2

3

1

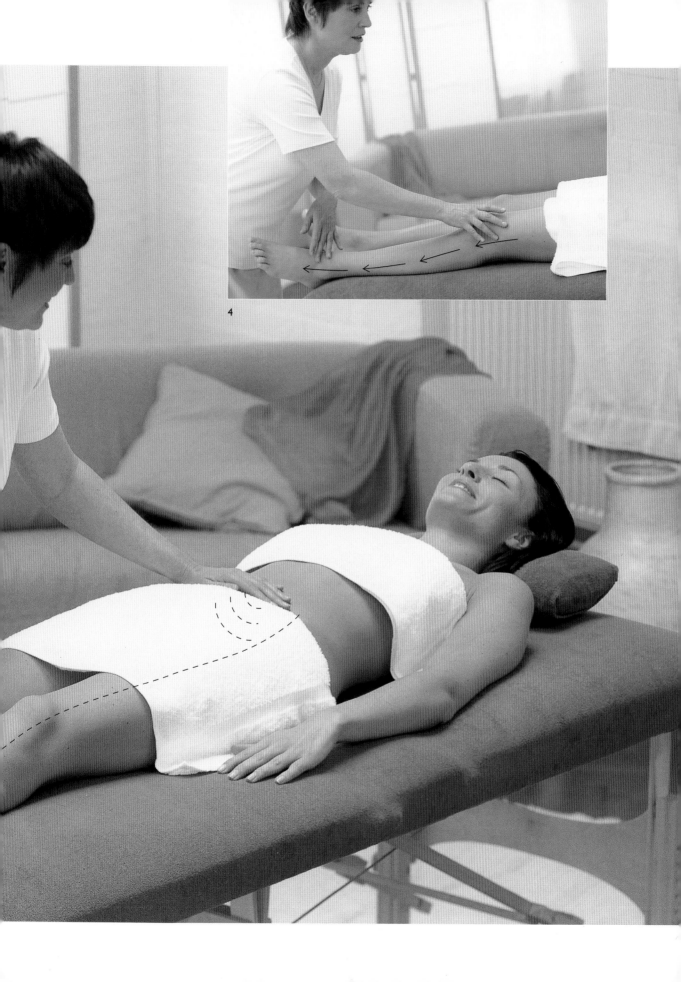

4

There are energy points in the feet. As they provide our contact with the ground, it is important that both muscles and joints are relaxed. By this stage your partner should be experiencing their body as one connected whole. However, ending the massage is as important as beginning. You have been working closely with your partner, both physically and mentally. Both of you have relaxed barriers and become more open, which is part of the healing process. However, to prevent your partner feeling vulnerable, it is important to provide a formal ending, reduce sensitivity and make a clear separation between you.

Step 1
Place one hand over the sole of the foot and flex the ankle by pressing back in line with the leg.

Step 2
Place both hands over the foot and spread your thumbs apart.

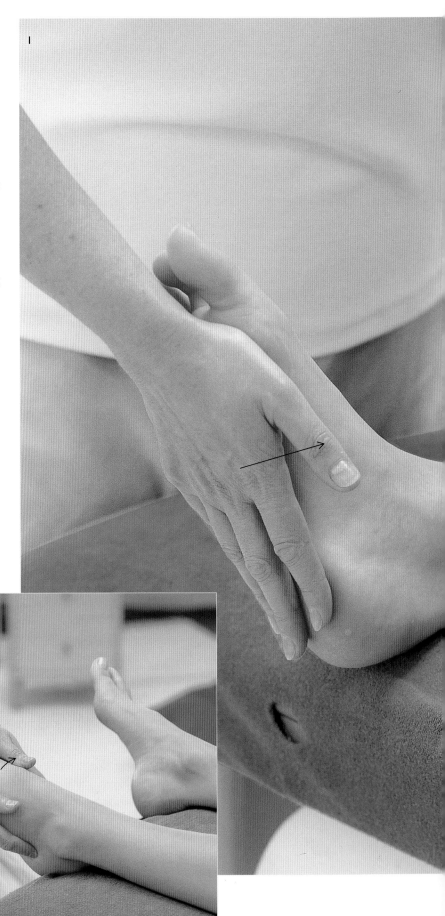

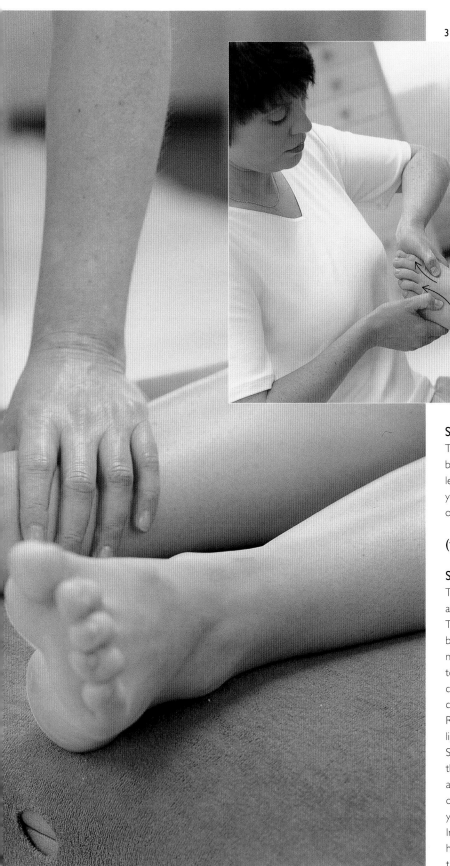

Step 3

To clear tension, draw downwards
between the toes and stroke the
length of the leg. End by drawing
your fingers over the toes. Repeat
on the other leg.

(for following see pages 98–99)

Step 4

The final connecting stroke focuses
attention on the entire body.
Throughout the massage, tension has
been released over various areas but
now is the time to draw the process
together. This technique, which is
called balancing, can also serve to
close down or reduce sensitivity.
Reach over and place your hands
lightly on the centre of the forehead.
Sweep around the head and down
the centre of the body to the
abdomen. Continue the movement
over both legs and end by placing
your hands over the soles of the feet.
Imagine energy coming through your
hands. When you are ready, gently
take them away.

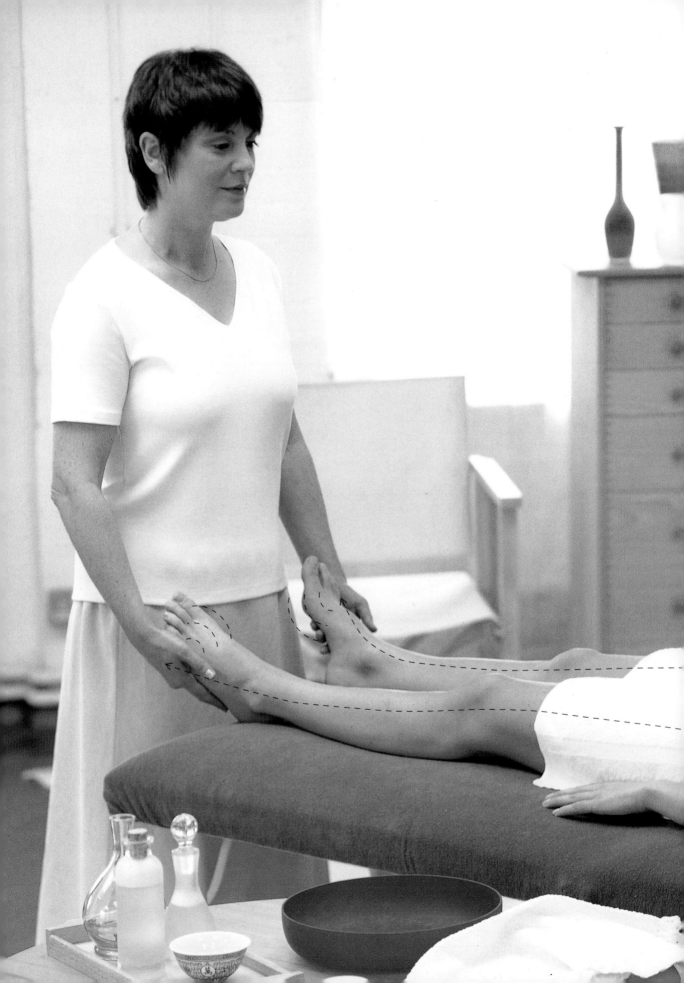

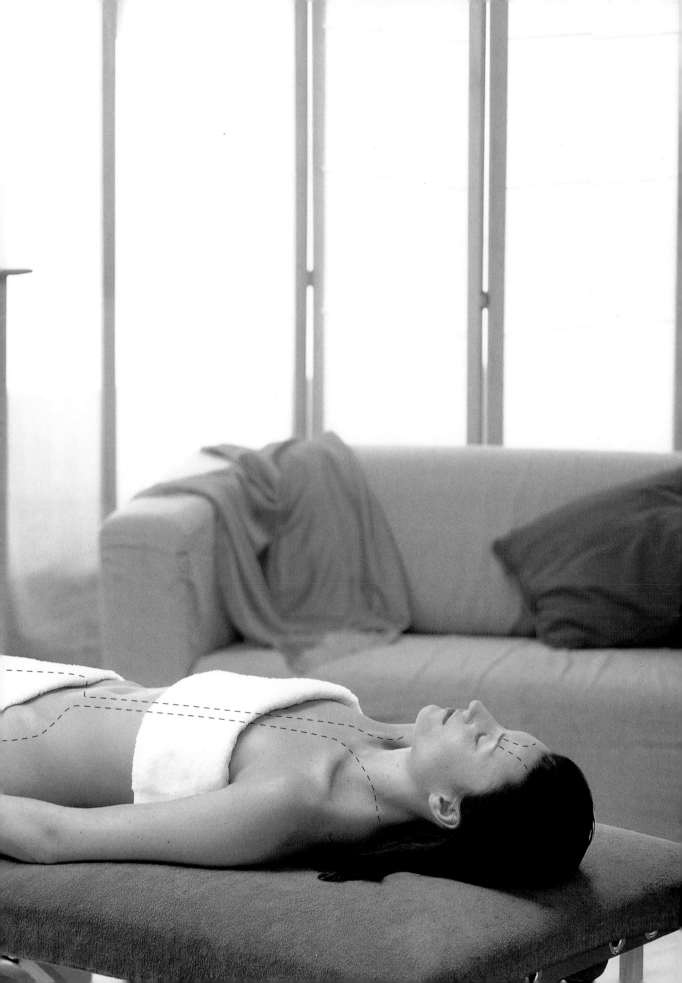

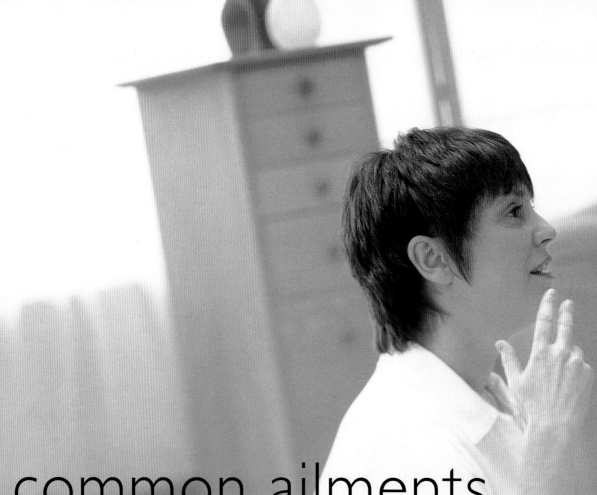

common ailments

The aim of any massage is to promote balance
and relaxation. Relaxation is vital in the healing
process and maximizes the body's restorative
powers. Bodily discomfort can signal that we are
under stress and, although a full healing massage
treats the whole body, if particular problems
cause distress it is helpful to concentrate on
specific areas. Before you begin, read the clues
your partner's body gives you. If you become
stuck, just relax and perform some simple strokes
until inspiration comes. Keep your mind going
forward as you work and don't try for immediate
results. These often come later. Finally, you
should be aware that you can only stimulate
self-healing – the rest is up to your partner.

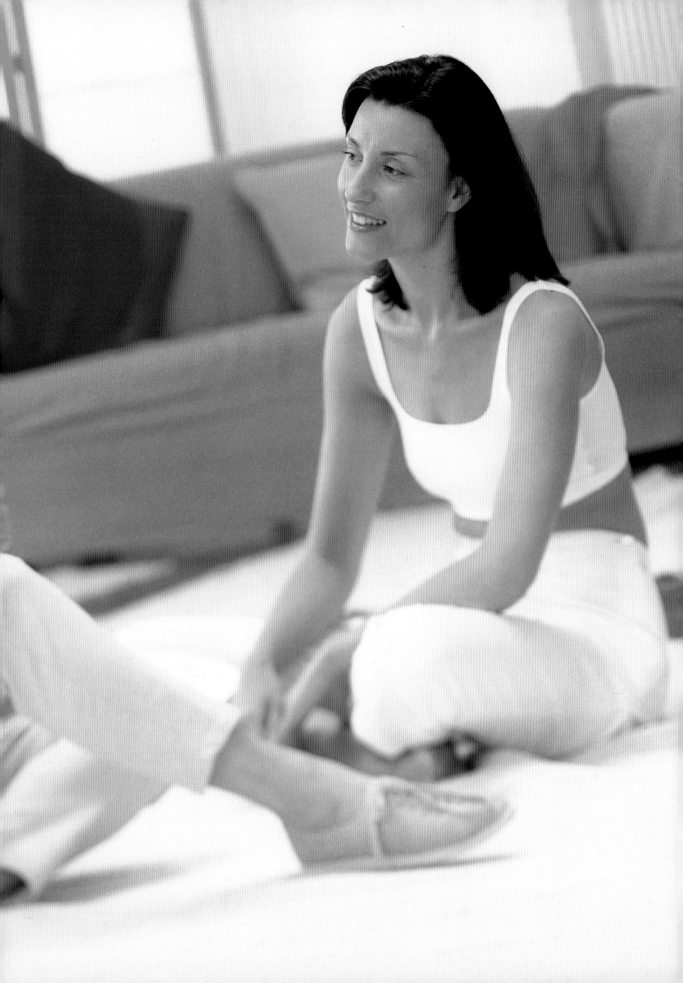

mind & brain

The nervous system is responsible for the way we interact with our environment. Stimuli, or incoming information, is received and processed and results in our response. The nervous system also regulates processes such as digestion, heart rate and breath. When it becomes overstimulated, the response is simply to shut down in order to reduce the overload. This is protection rather than illness and the process is a response to what we call stress. Such stress is responsible for a variety of states, such as anxiety, lethargy, depression, loss of self-esteem, and can result in muscular tension, headaches and acute sensitivity.

Stress

Try the techniques on page 103.

Loss of libido

Try the following techniques:
- Circle the lower abdomen to relax.
- Sweep diagonally across the abdomen to relax and increase sensation.
- Circle the upper thighs and hips with the heels of the hands to ease tension and increase sensation.
- Fan across the chest to soothe the heart and emotions.

Insomnia

Try the following techniques:
- Knead the upper back and shoulders to reduce tension and anxiety.
- Circle your thumbs over the soles of the feet to sedate.

Depression

Try the following techniques:
- Make small circles in a line from the forehead to the crown to lift the spirits.
- Make large circles over the upper back for comfort.
- Hold your hands above the abdomen and think positively. This helps to reduce mental stress.

'The majority of people who come for massage are suffering from stress in one form or another. It is such an overused word, however, and relaxation sounds so simple, that to my mind they do little to convey the sense of desperation some people feel. Learning to relax is one of the hardest things to do. I remember one woman who clearly appreciated massage and thoroughly enjoyed it, too. However, her conclusion was that ultimately it was no good. The reason? "It is addictive – you always want more!"'

Stress

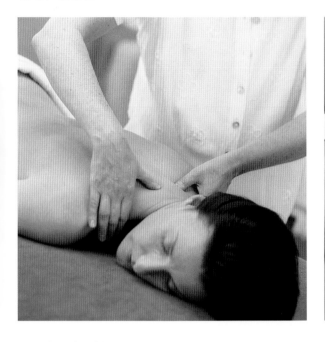

Kneading shoulders
Press, circle and squeeze the upper back muscles with your thumbs. Work up and down the muscles to the side of the spine to relieve the sense of pressure.

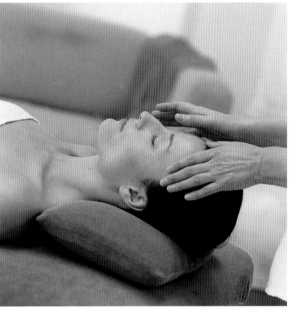

Stroking forehead
To de-stress and relax the eyes and forehead, gently stroke up the centre of the forehead with your thumbs. The effect should feel like rippling water.

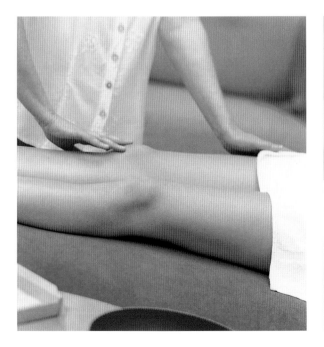

Stroking legs
To relax the lower body, gently stroke the length of the leg. Start from the hip and work down to the toe. Repeat several times on one leg, then on the other.

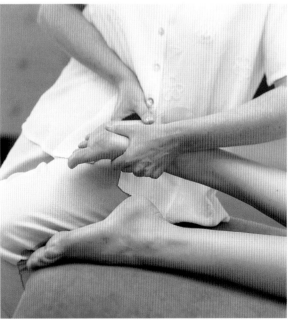

Stroking feet
Press and circle over the sole of the foot. Then stroke the foot, starting from the heel and working down to the toe. This will relax and soothe your partner.

mind & brain II

Headaches

Try the techniques on page 105.

Eyestrain

Try the following techniques:
- Draw firmly over the eyebrows to release tension above the eyes.
- Press firmly along the lower eye socket ridge to relax.
- Hold the hands over the eyes to rest.

Migraine

Try the following techniques before or after the onset of migraine:
- Knead across the top of the shoulders and base of the neck to relax.
- Gently press under the base of the skull with your thumb to release pressure.
- Gently rotate your fingers over the scalp to increase circulation.

Headache at the front of the head

Try the following techniques:
- Circle the temples to soothe.
- Make small, light circles over the forehead with your fingers to relax.
- Press firmly over the forehead to release tension.
- Press the web of the hand between finger and thumb to clear congestion.

Headache at the back of the head

Try the following techniques:
- Circle from the base of the neck to the skull for relaxation.
- Firmly rotate over the head to stimulate circulation.
- Press up the centre of the head towards the crown to relieve pain.

'Most clients suffer from headaches that are caused by bad posture and stress. As they learn to relax, so the headaches gradually decrease. But this is not always the case. One young man suffering from bad headaches had a terminal illness which remained undiagnosed until it had reached an advanced stage. He was very aware of the healing aspects of the massage as I worked over his head, and although at that stage there was nothing anyone could do, it at least helped him to relax and provided temporary relief. I remember him fondly.'

common ailments

Headaches

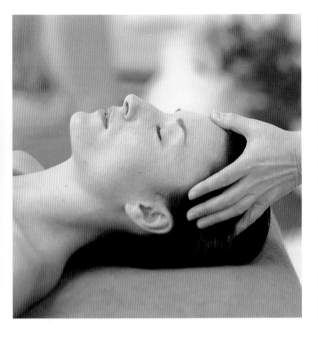

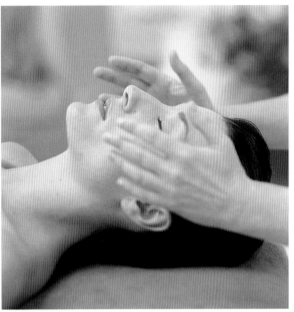

Pressing forehead

Place both thumbs in the centre of the forehead, just below the hairline. Press and release the thumbs, working in a line up to the centre of the head.

Circling head

Bring your hands to within 12–15 cm/5–6 inches of the head, or until you feel a tingling sensation. Make large, slow, circular movements towards you. Imagine that you are dissolving the pain.

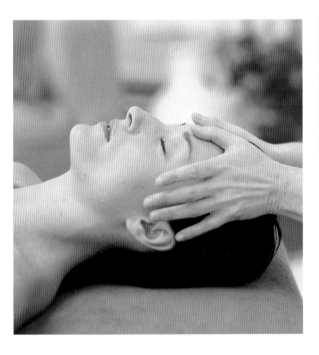

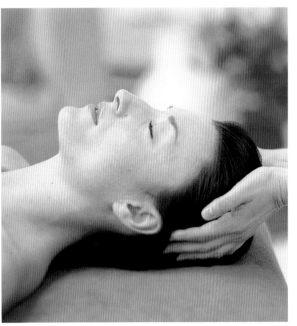

Sliding across forehead

Draw your thumbs across the forehead to soothe and release tension. Then repeat the movements slowly with your thumbs placed a 5 cm/2 inches above the head.

Holding head

Cup your hands around the back of the head. Just rest and relax. Imagine soothing energy is being released through your hands. Remain for several minutes.

respiration

The respiratory system is governed by the autonomic nervous system. As well as taking in air, the lungs are one of the main organs of elimination. They are concerned with the intake, assimilation and distribution of oxygen as a source of energy, and are affected by our environment as well as our nervous and emotional states. This is why, when we are under threat, our rate of respiration increases. Deep breathing, which involves the diaphragm and lower abdomen, makes us breathe properly and uses the majority of the lungs. Coughs, colds, asthma, hay fever and bronchitis are some of the common symptoms of respiratory stress.

Shallow breathing

Try the techniques on page 107.

Try the techniques on page 107.

Sinus

Try the following techniques:
- Press under the cheekbones to ease away pressure.
- Press to the sides of the nose to help relieve congestion.
- Press up the centre of the forehead to relax tension.

Coughs

Try the following techniques:
- Cup your hands over the upper back to relieve congestion.
- Press your thumbs between the upper ribs to calm.

Head cold

Try the following techniques:
- Press the web of skin between finger and thumb to relieve congestion.
- Press between the eyebrows to help relieve pressure.
- Press into the muscles at the sides of the spine over the upper back to promote relaxation.

'The way we breathe says a lot about how relaxed we are. Sometimes it takes a bit of practice. Recently, one of my clients was suffering from anxiety, feeling negative about life and having bad dreams. Her breathing was tense, even when lying down, and she almost seemed to be holding her breath. I suggested some simple exercises which she practises night and morning, and she is gradually starting to feel better.'

Shallow breathing

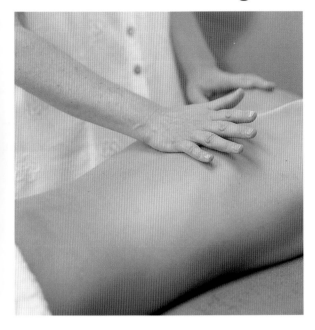

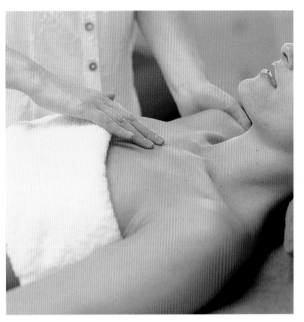

Circling back
Place your hand between the shoulder blades and make large slow circles over the upper back, moving in an anticlockwise direction. This helps to soothe and relax.

Stroking chest
To relax the upper chest, gently stroke downwards with the thumbs and fingers. Imagine you are calming and inducing a sense of relaxation through the body.

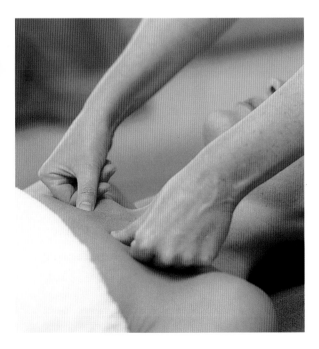

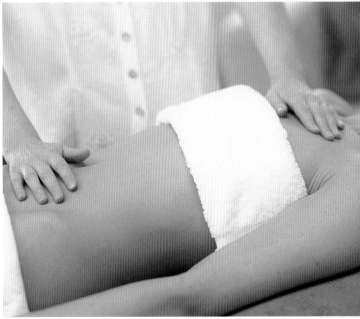

Pressing ribs
Lean over your partner and place your thumbs between the ribs, to either side of the breastbone. Press and release evenly to relieve tension.

Balancing upper/lower body
Place one hand lightly over the upper chest and the other over the lower abdomen. Simply rest while the body relaxes and breathing becomes deeper.

circulation

The circulatory system is governed by the autonomic nervous system. As with our breathing rate, the sympathetic nervous system is responsible for an increase in heart rate when we need to take action or are under stress. The lymphatic system, which plays a major role in the body's immune responses, arises from the vascular system. Massage aids circulation by helping drain muscle tissues and assists the return of the blood supply to the heart. Poor circulation, high and low blood pressure, palpitations and varicose veins are some of the problems that can arise. Massage can reduce stress in cases of high blood pressure or a heart condition, but you must seek your doctor's advice first.

Circulation

Try the techniques on page 109.

High blood pressure

Try the following techniques:
- Effleurage lightly over the body to encourage relaxation.
- Gently circle the temples to help ease stress.

Puffy ankles

Try the following techniques:
- Circle around the affected area to increase circulation.
- Apply pressure upwards over the calf to assist drainage.

Palpitations

Try the following techniques:
- Stroke down the front of the body to calm the system.
- Stroke over the forehead to help reduce anxiety.

'I always work cautiously when someone has a heart condition, but as long as their doctor has given approval, massage really seems to help. It can ease the stress of waiting for surgery and aid the recovery process. A hospital told one of my clients that they wished massage could be provided for all their patients. Another client embarked on massage as part of a programme to reduce his blood pressure. It returned to normal after several weeks.'

Circulation

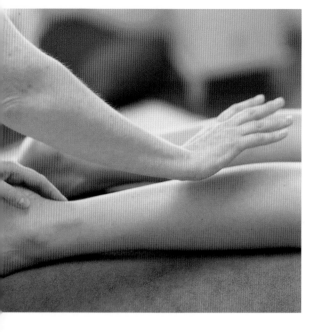

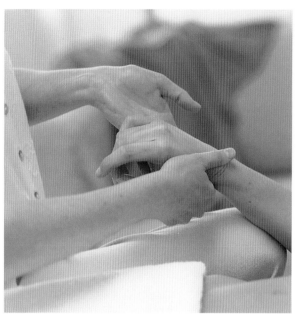

Brushing varicose veins

Avoid pressure over varicose veins by holding your hands 5 cm/2 inches from the leg and brushing upwards over the affected area. Repeat several times, stroking towards the heart.

Draining cold hands

Rub and shake the hands and squeeze the fingers to warm them, then press and drain upwards over the hand to stimulate circulation. Work towards the wrist.

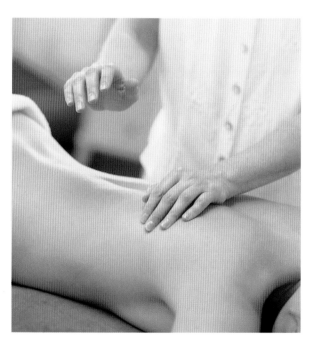

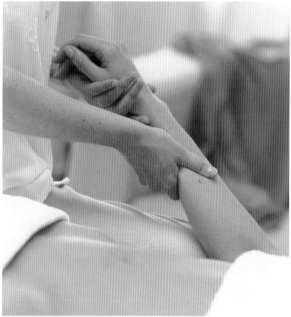

Cupping back

Use cupping movements to stimulate the circulation in the back. Cup your hands and then tap quickly and lightly. Avoid working on the spine itself.

Draining arm

Support the arm and squeeze over the muscles, working towards the elbow, in the direction of the heart. Use pressure with fingers and thumb to stimulate muscle drainage.

digestion

Digestive processes are governed by the autonomic nervous system. The digestive system functions properly when the body is at ease but, when we are under stress, the abdominal blood supply is reduced. Digestion is put on hold and tightness, sensitivity and burning pains are felt around the solar plexus. Digestion involves the absorption and distribution of nutrients. Inability to assimilate these nutrients results in diarrhoea and may cause constipation. Ulcers, heartburn, flatulence, irritable bowel syndrome and fatigue are other problems that may arise. Ideally, the abdomen should be naturally relaxed and full, rather than held in – very different from the way we are usually taught to hold our bodies.

Digestive problems

Try the techniques on page 111.

Stomach ache

Try the following techniques:
- Hold your hand 5 cm/2 inches away from the stomach to relieve pain.
- Circle the abdomen to relieve tension.

Bloating

Try the following techniques:
- Sweep diagonally to ease discomfort.
- Lightly hand press under the ribs to aid digestion.
- Gently effleurage over the stomach to calm and soothe.

Constipation

Try the following techniques:
- Press in the web between first finger and thumb to stimulate elimination.
- Firmly effleurage and make small fingertip circles over the lower abdomen to encourage relaxation.

'The mind can play strange tricks. One day I was massaging one of my clients and had just finished working over his head and face. He seemed blissfully relaxed. However, when I moved to his side and began massaging his abdomen, I saw him squinting at me out of the corner of his eye. When I asked if everything was all right, he replied he was absolutely fine, only a bit puzzled as he could still feel my hands on his head.'

Digestive problems

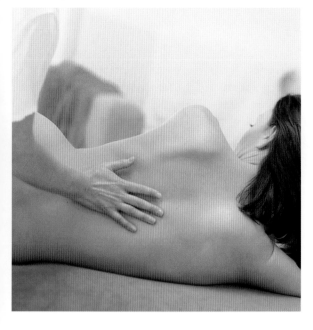

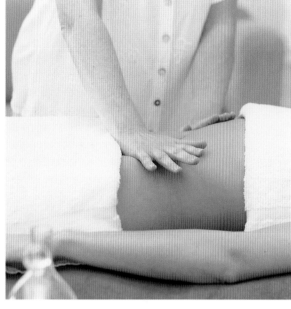

Circling back
Using the flat of your hands, make large circles over the middle of the back. Circle in an anticlockwise direction, making the movements as soothing as possible.

Diagonal sweep across abdomen
Place both hands over the abdomen and then draw them diagonally apart towards the ribcage and hip. Keep your hands flat and repeat more firmly. Repeat the opposite way.

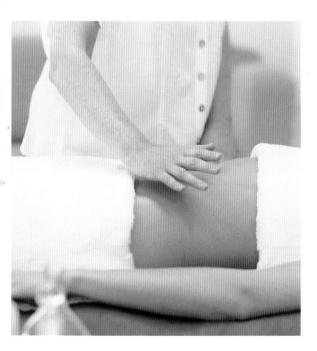

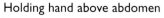

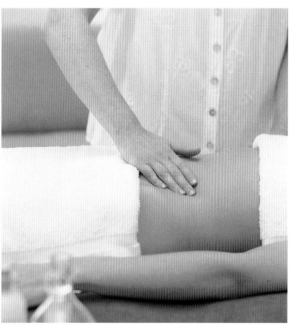

Holding hand above abdomen
To ease pain, hold your hand 5 cm/2 inches above the lower abdomen. Imagine you are releasing stress and congestion. Release when you feel a change.

Small circles over abdomen
Move over the lower abdomen in a clockwise circle, making a series of smaller circles with your fingers. Repeat the circles over tense areas to help them relax.

reproduction

It will come as no surprise that the reproductive system, not being a priority in the face of imminent danger, also suffers from a reduced blood supply when under stress. Governed by the autonomic nervous system, reproductive health is affected by emotional stability and physical well-being. Menstrual pains, missed periods, premenstrual tension (PMT), lack of sex drive and menopausal distress are some of the most common problems. Massage prior to, and during, pregnancy is perfectly safe and can help reduce water retention and discomfort in the later stages. However, never use any stimulating strokes, always massage gently and avoid working over the abdomen during the first four months.

Menstrual pains and PMT

Try the techniques on page 113.

Menopausal discomfort

Try the following techniques:
- Drain the calves and thighs to reduce fluid retention.
- Knead the hips and thighs to stimulate muscle drainage.
- Effleurage over the skin with nourishing oil to combat dryness.

Pregnancy

Try the following techniques
- Gently effleurage the entire back to relieve strain and discomfort.
- Thumb spread over the top of the feet to relieve aches.
- Stroke the hands and temples to soothe and induce relaxation.
- Rest your hands lightly over the abdomen to offer support.

Water retention

Try the following techniques:
- Circle clockwise over the abdomen to ease bloating.
- Circle anticlockwise over the lower back to stimulate elimination.

'Necessity is a great teacher! A friend's sister was lying on the sofa clutching a hot water bottle and yelping with menstrual cramps. Circling her lower back gradually brought relief and has now become a standard. However, you have to drop all the rules during pregnancy. One friend could not find a comfortable position. It took a lot of cushions, ingenuity and the floor to find a position that ultimately worked for her.'

Menstrual pains and PMT

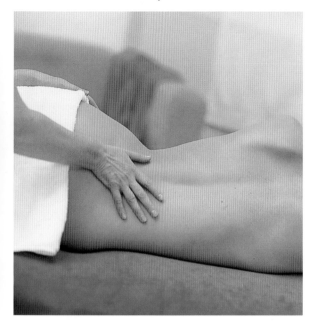

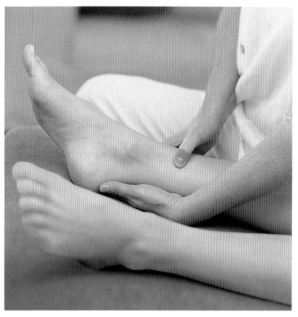

Circling back
Circle your hands anticlockwise over the lower back and sacrum to relieve period pains. The warmth of your hands will help the relaxation process.

Pressing ankle
To relieve PMT and menstrual pains, place your hand roughly three finger widths up from the top of the ankle and press your thumb over the bone. *Do not use if you are pregnant.*

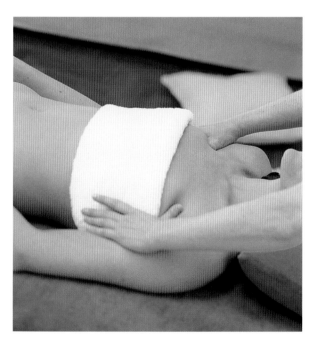

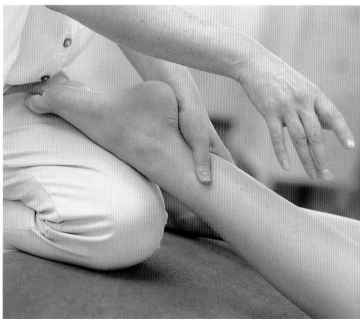

Draining across chest
To ease swollen breasts, draw your thumbs across the top of the chest and drain down towards the armpits. Avoid pressing over any tender areas.

Draining leg
To ease water retention, stimulate drainage of the muscles by squeezing upwards from the ankle and over the calf. Apply pressure between fingers and thumb.

muscular pain

The skeletal muscles, those within our conscious control, are governed by the central nervous system. Stimuli are transmitted to the spinal cord and brain while impulses for movement and activity are received via the peripheral nerves. Waste products are carried away by the venous and lymph systems. Prolonged contraction affects the drainage of the muscles and reduces the mobility of the joints. When we are under stress there may be localized numbness or loss of sensation. Our muscles, and hence our body shape, reflect our continual process of metabolism. Back pain, repetitive strain injury, frozen shoulder, painful joints, sciatica and headaches are some of the associated problems.

Neck and shoulders

Try the techniques on page 115.

Lower back stress

Try the following techniques:
○ Sweep diagonally across the muscles to provide a stretch.
○ Press the muscles to the sides of the spine to relax.
○ Circle the lower back to encourage relaxation.

Mild sciatic pain

Try the following techniques:
○ Circle the sacrum to relax.
○ Thumb press and make small circles over the sacrum to relieve pain.
○ Knead carefully over the buttocks to improve circulation.

'Many people prefer to have a massage at the end of the day or week so that they can continue to relax afterwards. The problem for many people working long office hours is they feel they can't take the time to relax. One particular lady who runs her own business appreciates that stress slows you down, so she regularly nips in for a lunchtime massage, so she can sail through her afternoon meetings.'

Neck and shoulders

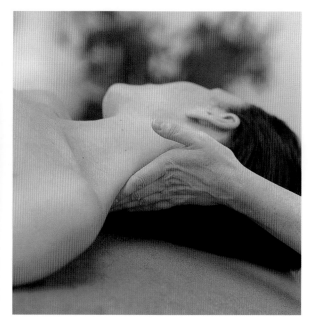

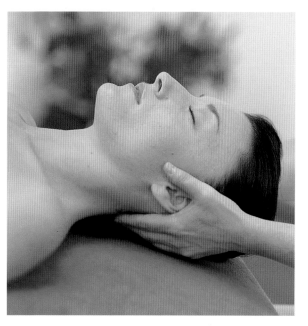

Clearing neck
Turn the head to one side, reach down under the shoulder with your other hand and draw your fingers up alongside the spine to the base of the skull.

Pulling neck
Place both hands securely beneath the neck. Lift the head slightly and gently pull it towards you, letting your hands slide up to the base of the skull.

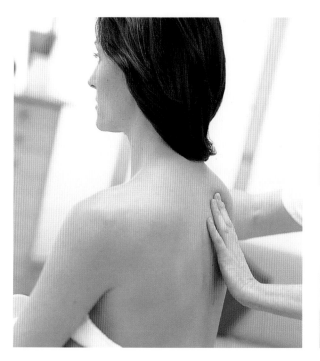

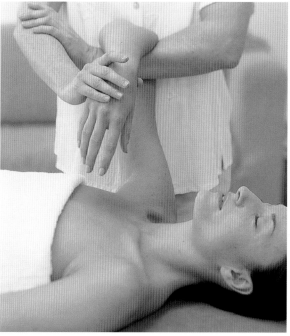

Press shoulder
Support the front of the shoulder with one hand, then press around the line of the shoulder blade with fingers and thumb. Press firmly in towards the blade.

Arm lift
Crook your partner's arm over your own, hold the wrist with your other hand and then gently pull the arm first towards you, then upwards. Repeat slowly.

muscular pain II

Ankle sprain

Try the techniques on page 117.

Repetitive strain injury

Try the following techniques:
- Effleurage and knead around the shoulder to relax the muscles.
- Thumb spread gently over the forearm to reduce tension.
- Press over the hand and draw between the fingers to ease muscle contraction.

Facial tension

Try the following techniques:
- Stroke between the brows to soften the appearance.
- Draw over the cheeks to encourage relaxation.
- Circle the temples to reduce irritability.

Aching feet

Try the following techniques:
- Thumb spread over the foot to relax the muscles.
- Circle the ankles to aid circulation.
- Press over the soles of the feet to reduce tiredness.

Cramp

Try the following techniques:
- Knead the calf muscles to ease the contraction.
- Press firmly over the sole of the foot to reduce spasm.

Stiff hips

Try the following techniques:
- Knead the hips and buttocks to increase circulation.
- Press around the hip joint to relax the muscles.

'One woman had broken her ankle on a skiing holiday. After weeks in plaster followed by physiotherapy, she felt there was more progress to be made. Working first above her ankle and then, as she grew stronger, around and on it, she experienced deep sensations of tingling and re-experienced some of the pain. She is still regaining movement and sensation and regularly experiences "healing spurts".'

Ankle sprain

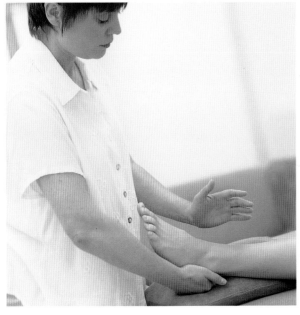

Circling ankle
Hold your hand above the ankle. Note the sensations and then draw your hand away. Make small circles above the affected area, then repeat still further away.

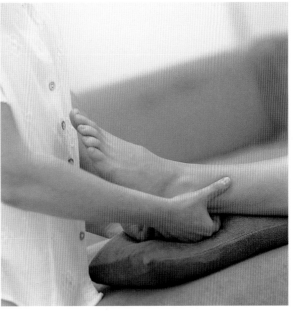

Draining leg
Support the foot. Press upwards over the leg to stimulate drainage, always working above the swelling. Work gently. If the skin is red, begin higher up.

Stroking ankle
Hold your hand a 5 cm/2 inches above the ankle. Gently stroke towards the foot and over the toes. Imagine you are helping to soothe inflammation.

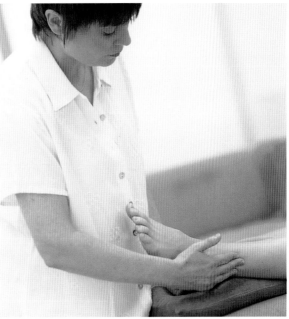

Pressing ankle
Support the foot and then make small circular movements around – but not over – the site of the swelling. This will help to reduce pain and drain fluids.

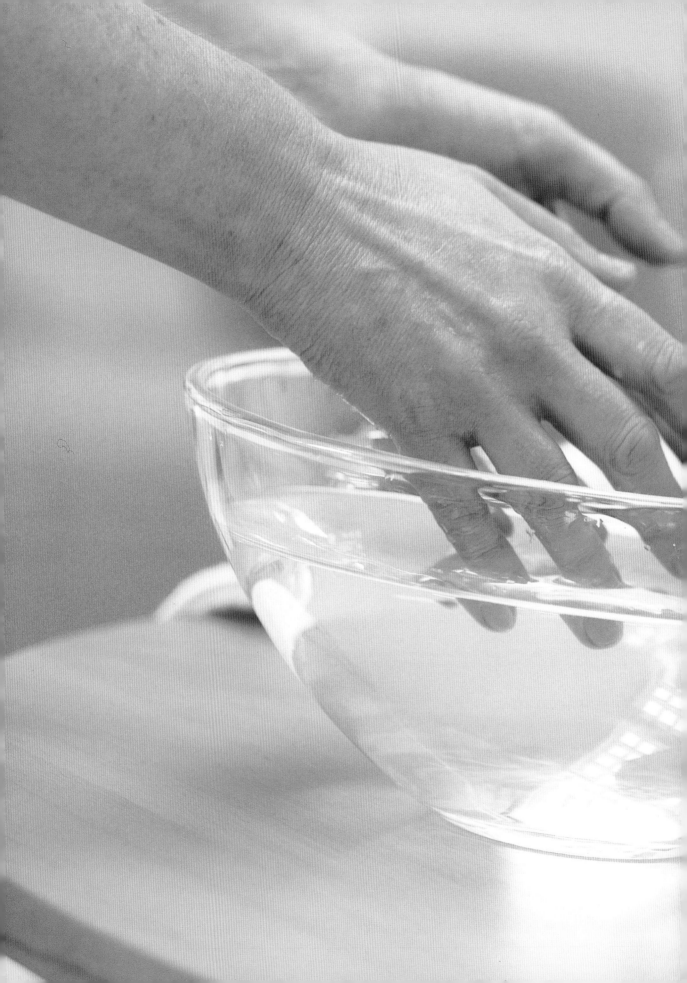

self healing

An important part of the healing process is learning to take care of ourselves. Self healing can become part of our daily routine to relax and maintain our health or treat minor ailments. Self healing provides an opportunity to experiment, make discoveries and gain valuable confidence. Healing is about learning, so trust your body's signals and find out what works for you. It is all too easy to focus on other people and forget about our own needs. Relaxing mind and body, developing interests and taking responsibility for ourselves and what happens to us is essential for our health, happiness and growth.

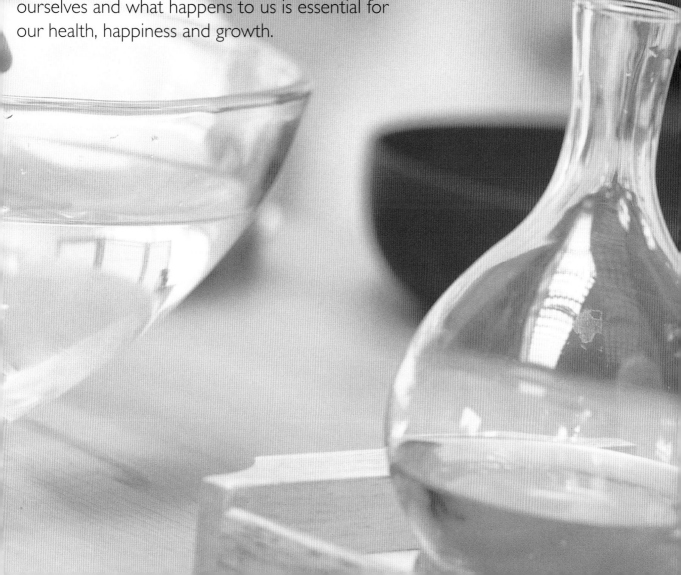

We all have the power within to heal ourselves. When we go to see someone else for help we are usually depleted or perhaps confused about what to do or what is wrong. When another person works with us, this helps to restore our confidence and activates our ability for self healing. We can make use of the input provided by the other person and of their knowledge, which may be greater than ours. Working with another person can also help us to achieve a better state of clarity when we are ill or going round in circles. However, healing is ultimately about self healing. With a few exceptions, nobody else can actually do it for us. Whether we are interested in working with other people or just in maintaining health in our everyday lives, we need to get to know ourselves a little better and help ourselves more often. It is a question of listening to what our bodies tell us, of actually being still and listening, instead of the constant rush we all get caught up in. Working on ourselves is also helpful for learning and practising techniques, finding out which ones work for us and which don't. We can then use this information when we work with other people.

Here are some very straightforward techniques to work on the vital energy field. These will energize and uplift or sedate. Tension headaches, which are a common problem for most of us, can be relieved by a gentle massage followed by dispersal techniques which draw pain away from the body and change our mood.

self healing

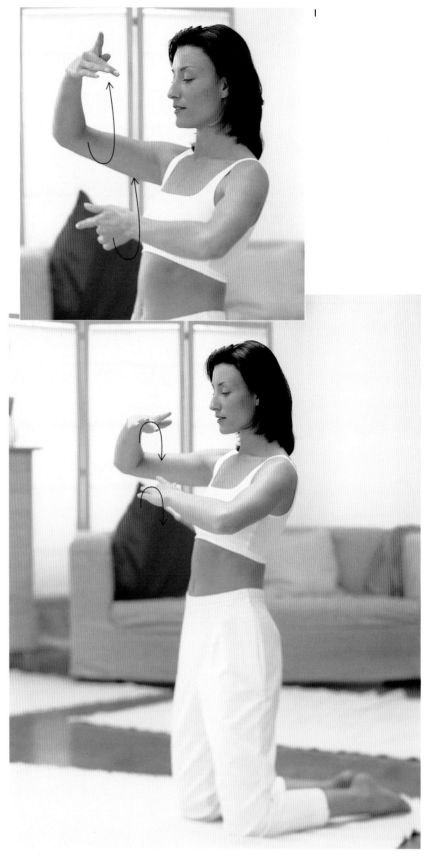

I

2

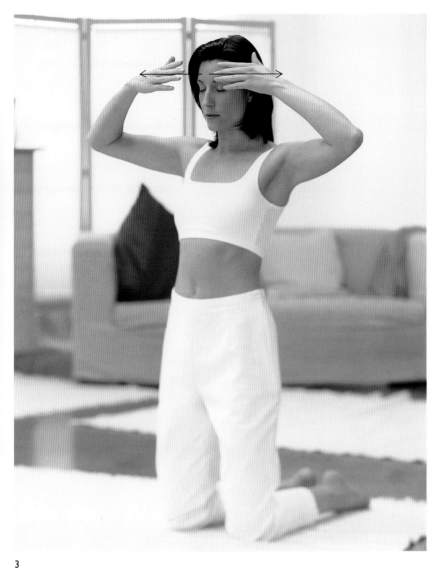

1 Brushing up

To energize and lift your spirits, hold your hands about 20–25 cm/ 8–10 inches away from your body. Begin by brushing your hands upwards from the top of the chest, continuing up over the face and head. The hands perform the movements alternately in quick, light succession.

2 Brushing down

To relax and sedate, perform the movements the opposite way, beginning at the top of the head and stroking downwards. This time your hands should be heavier and should move more slowly. Repeat the movements rhythmically over the face to the top of the chest, keeping your hands at the same distance.

3 Drawing across the forehead

To help relieve a tension headache and relax, first work over the forehead with physical strokes. Then hold your hands roughly 10–12 cm/4–5 inches away from your forehead. Note the sensations in your hands as well as the way your headache responds. Try to get a sense of engaging the pain.

4 Drawing away

Continue the movement by slowly drawing your hands apart over your forehead and continuing away from the head. Mould your movements to the shape of your head. Mentally relax as you do so. Imagine you are releasing all the tightness and pain. Repeat the strokes as necessary.

3

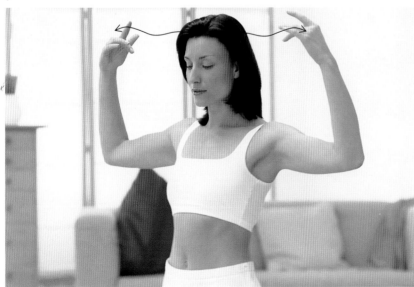

4

Taking the time to stop and centre ourselves, or 'tune in', each day is very important. It takes a bit of practice at first, but after a while it becomes routine. We should not be endlessly introverted or self-examining, but we do need to catch up with what goes on inside us – otherwise it will catch up with us instead. Giving ourselves several minutes of breathing space each day is vital to healthy living. In addition, applying massage and healing techniques and breathing calmly when we are feeling stressed relaxes both body and mind. Quietening the mind reduces mental stress, produces clearer thinking and avoids us spending nervous energy on endless thoughts. When you are practising techniques on yourself, concentrate your attention on the sensations you feel and make note of the things that make a difference. Begin the process with a purpose in mind, for example to relax your breathing. Notice what it is you usually do – for most of us it involves tension in the upper chest. Then, if you need to bring about a change, focus your attention further down. Very often our energies are unfocused or misdirected, and this affects the healing process. Whether working on yourself or another person, it is important to concentrate and think of them, or yourself, as being well. This type of visualization helps athletes to win races and similar techniques are used in the business world. After all, if we can't even imagine achieving something, how are we ever going to accomplish it?

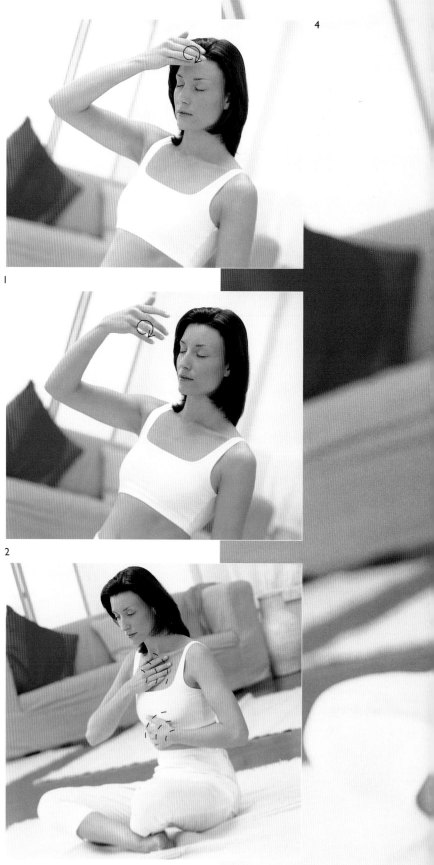

4

1

2

3

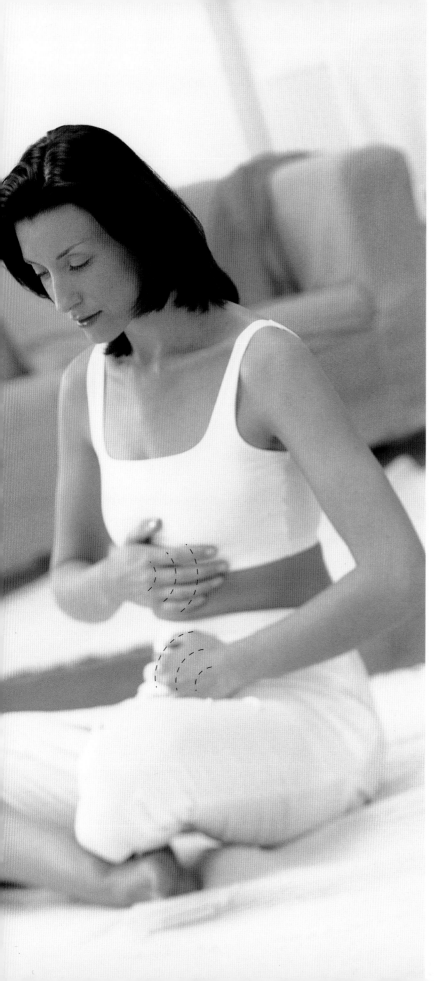

1 Circling forehead

To relieve a throbbing headache, first work over the head to encourage the muscles to relax. Then place your hand roughly 10–13 cm/4–5 inches away from the centre of your forehead. Try to engage the pain and make small circles moving slightly away from you.

2 Pulling away

With your hand in the same position, imagine you are drawing the pain away. Move your hand 5 cm/2 inches further away from your body and repeat the circling movements. Notice the difference this makes. Bring your hand closer once more and then further away. Continue until the pain eases.

3 Relaxed breathing (1)

Sit, stand or lie in a comfortable position. Place one hand over the top of your chest and the other over your solar plexus. Without trying, breathe naturally and notice the movement in your chest as you breathe. If you feel tense, just relax a bit more. Don't try to do anything. Just rest your hands and observe.

4 Relaxed breathing (2)

Place your upper hand over your lower abdomen, keeping the other hand where it is. Breathe naturally and focus your attention on the warmth coming from your hands. Don't try to do anything, simply notice if this feels any different. Concentrate on your hands and the gentle rhythm of your breath.

self healing

looking after yourself

As someone giving massage, there is probably one person to whom you pay the least attention – yourself. It is a curious thing, but people who take care of other people are absolutely the worst at taking care of themselves. If you give massage on a regular basis this amounts to little short of foolishness. You are all you've got! It is vital to look after yourself, keep fit and healthy and work to strengthen your abilities. To develop your skills and understanding I highly recommend regular relaxation, meditation and some physical work like yoga or a martial art. This will help keep your mind clear and give an edge to your massage work. After each massage you give you must pay some attention to yourself. Washing your hands is not only hygienic, it also helps avoid absorbing stress. It is always advisable to perform some form of cleansing techniques and take time to centre yourself. This will help to prevent 'burnout'. It also makes sense – and is extremely important – to receive massage regularly. At the very least it will keep reminding you how wonderful it actually feels. You will also be able to pick up new ideas. Massage is a physical skill where you deal with someone very closely and on quite subtle levels. This requires self-discipline and your full concentration while you work. It is a wonderful art to practise. To make sure it stays that way remember to relax often, switch off and have fun!

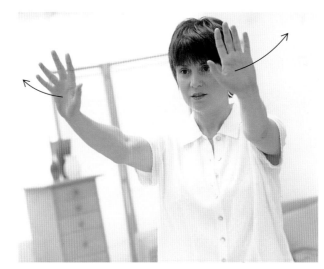

1

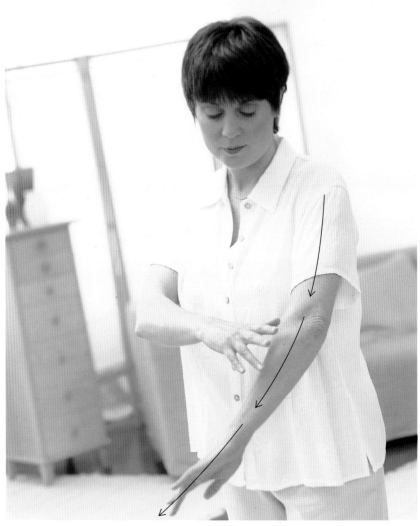

2

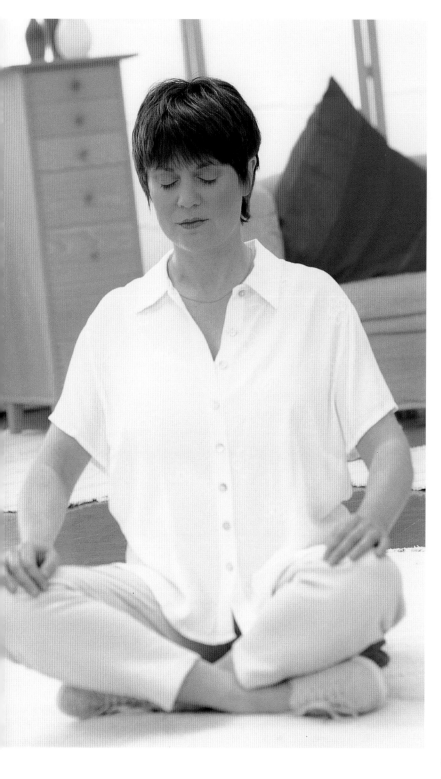

1 Clear around head

After each massage, wash your hands. To release any stress you may have picked up you need to clear your vital energy field. To do this, hold your hands in front of you and then push away with extended arms around your face, head and shoulders. Repeat the movements several times. It should feel like a breath of fresh air.

2 Clear arms

Continue the sequence by brushing downwards over both arms, then over the front of your body. Reach up behind your shoulder blades and brush down your back to the floor. Brush vigorously, with your hands a 5 cm/2 inches from your body, until you feel lighter and experience a change in feeling or mood.

Centring

To centre yourself, stand in a relaxed position with shoulders loose and feet firmly on the ground. Imagine you are relaxing from the top of your head to your feet. Actually feel it happening. As you do so, relax any nervous energy out through your feet. Concentrate on your contact with the ground.

Massage can do a tremendous amount of good. Just the time spent together focusing on the same experience is rare enough. Have confidence that your partner will benefit from the best you are capable of, and if you have any doubts, always say 'no'. When people are stressed or ill they can be difficult, so don't take things personally. A healing massage, performed with care and sensitivity, can make a real difference. Healing may inspire, change attitudes, help people through crisis and encourage growth. There is a point where you feel something flowing through you – just let go so the process can take place.

index

acknowledgements

Publishing Director: Alison Goff
Commissioning Editor: Jane McIntosh
Editors: Clare Hill and Catharine Davey
Creative Director: Keith Martin
Executive Art Editor: Mark Winward
Designer: Louise Griffiths
Photography: Peter Myers
Stylist: Penny Markham
Picture Research: Sally Claxton and Charlotte Deane
Production Controller: Dawn Mitchell

First published in Great Britain in 1997 by Hamlyn,
a division of Octopus Publishing Group Limited
2–4 Heron Quays, London E14 4JP

Reprinted 2001

Copyright © 1997, 2001 Octopus Publishing Group Limited
Text copyright © 1997 Susan Mumford

ISBN 0 600 60492 6

A CIP catalogue record of this book is available
on request.

Printed in Hong Kong

The publishers would like to thank Virgo Bodywork Tables, PO
Box 13835, London, N15 3WD for the loan of the massage
table and Tavy Covers for the loan of the covers.

The publishers would like to thank the following individuals and
organizations for their kind permission to reproduce
photographs in this book:
Octopus Publishing Group Ltd./Peter Myers 1, 2/3, 4/5, 8/9,
18/19, 20/1, 22 BL, 22 T, 23 T, 23 B, 24 T, 24 B, 25 T, 25 B, 26 T,
26 B, 27 T, 27 B, 28 T, 28 B, 29 T, 29 B, 30 , 31 T, 31 B, 32/3, 33
BR, 34 , 35 , 36 B, 36/7, 37 T, 37 B, 38 T, 38 B, 39 T, 39 B, 40 T,
40 B, 41 T, 41 B, 42 T, 42 B, 43 T, 43 B, 44/5, 45 inset, 46/7, 46
BL 46 BR, 46 T, 47 T, , 48 T, 48 B, 49 , 50 T, 50 B, 51 T, 51 B, 51
C, 52, 53, 54, 55 , 56 , 57 B, 57 T, 58 T, 60, 61, 62/3, 64/65 (1),
64 inset bottom (2), 65 inset top (3), 65 inset centre right (4),
66 T, 66 C, 66 B, 67 T,67 C, 67 B, 68 T, 68 B, 68/9, 69 T, 69
B,70/1, 70 B, 71 T, 71 B, 72/3, 73 T, 73 B, 74 T, 74 B, 75 T, 75 B,
76 T, 76 B, 77 T, 77 C, 77 B, 78 B, 78/9, 79 TL, 79 TR, 80 T, 80
C, 80 B, 81 T, 81 B, 82 T, 82 C, 82 B, 83 T, 83 B, 84 B, 84/5, 85
T, 86 B, 86/7, 87 T, 88 B, 88/9, 89 T, 89 B, 90 T, 90/1, 91, 92 T,
92 B, 93 T, 93 B, 94 T, 94 B, 94/5, 95 T, 96 B, 96/7, 97, 98/99,
100/1, 103 TL, 103 TR, 103 BL, 103 BR, 105 TL, 105 TR, 105
BL,105 BR, 107 TL, 107 TR, 107 BL, 107 BR, 109 TL, 109 TR,
109 BL, 109 BR, 111 TL, 111 TR, 111 BL, 111 BR, 113 TL, 113
TR, 113 BL, 113 BR, 115 TL, 115 TR, 115 BL, 115 BR, 117 TL,
117 TR, 117 BL, 117 BR, 118/9, 120 T, 120 B, 121 T, 121 B, 122
T, 122 C, 122 B, 123, 124 T, 124 B, 125
AKG London 17
Science Photo Library/G. Hadjo, CNRI 11

author's acknowledgements

Sincere thanks to Jane McIntosh, Louise Griffiths, Catharine Davey and Keith Martin at Octopus. Thanks
also to my agent, Mandy Little. Many thanks to photographer Peter Myers and assistant Sean Myers, to
Andrea Black for makeup and model Danielle Walsh.

My thanks once again to W. Llewellyn McKone, DO, MRO, Lecturer in Osteopathic Sports Medicine, and
Ken Lloyd, President of the Register of Chinese Herbal Medicine. I would like to thank my massage
teachers, particularly Sara Thomas, and more recently Steve Bird, Barbara Simons and Eve Taylor. Thanks
also to the National Federation of Spiritual Healers, and teachers at the British T'ai Chi Ch'uan
Association and Marpa House.